NURSING PROCESS SUMMARY

Assessment. Collecting and recording data to provide the information needed to:

- [ ] Predict, detect, prevent, manage, or eliminate health problems.
- [ ] Predict, detect, prevent, manage, or eliminate risk factors.
- [ ] Clarify expected outcomes (measurable expected results or benefits of care).
- [ ] Identify interventions to achieve outcomes, promote health, and attain optimum function and independence.

Diagnosis. Analyzing and synthesizing data to draw conclusions to:

- [ ] Identify signs and symptoms that may indicate the need for referral to a more qualified professional (report these immediately).
- [ ] Identify patterns; generate a list of suspected problems that need to be ruled out.
- [ ] Clarify actual and potential health problems and underlying contributing factors.
- [ ] Identify risk (related) factors.
- [ ] Determine resources, strengths, use of healthy behaviors
- [ ] Recognize health states that could be improved.
- [ ] Ensure learning, communication, and safety needs are identified.
- [ ] **Reflect on thinking** to determine whether: (1) patient participation in the process has been at an optimum level, (2) data is accurate and complete, (3) assumptions have been identified; (4) conclusions are based on facts (evidence), rather than guesswork, and (5) alternate conclusions, ideas, and solutions have been considered. (This applies to *all the phases*, but is placed here because it requires analysis, which is the focus of this phase.)

Planning. Ensuring that the patient has an individualized, comprehensive plan by clarifying expected outcomes, individualizing interventions, and making sure the plan is adequately recorded. The plan should be designed to:

- [ ] Detect, prevent, and manage the health problems and their underlying contributing factors.
- [ ] Focus on priority problems and risk factors (those that *must* be managed to achieve the overall outcomes of care).
- [ ] Promote optimum function, independence, and well-being.
- [ ] Coordinate care and include patients as partners in decision making and care.
- [ ] Achieve the desired outcomes safely, efficiently, and cost-effectively.
- [ ] Provide teaching to help patients make informed decisions.
- [ ] Make a record that can be used to monitor progress and communicate care.

Implementation. Putting the plan into action by:

- [ ] Assessing appropriateness of interventions and deciding whether the patient is ready
- [ ] Prioritizing, delegating, and coordinating care as indicated, including patients as partners in decision making
- [ ] Preparing the environment and equipment for safety, comfort, and convenience
- [ ] Performing interventions, then reassess to determine initial responses
- [ ] Making immediate changes as needed
- [ ] Charting to monitor progress and communicate care
- [ ] Updating the plan as needed

Evaluation.

- [ ] Assess patient status to determine whether expected outcomes have been met and what factors promoted or inhibited the success of the plan.
- [ ] Plan for ongoing assessment, improvement, and patient independence.
- [ ] Discharge the patient or modifying the plan as indicated.

Applying Nursing Process

The Foundation for Clinical Reasoning

8th Edition

Rosalinda Alfaro-LeFevre, RN, MSN, ANEF

President
Teaching Smart/Learning Easy
Stuart, Florida
www.AlfaroTeachSmart.com

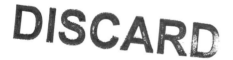
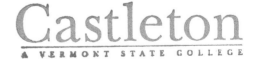

Castleton
A VERMONT STATE COLLEGE

Wolters Kluwer | Lippincott Williams & Wilkins
Health
Philadelphia · Baltimore · New York · London
Buenos Aires · Hong Kong · Sydney · Tokyo

Acquisitions Editor: Patrick Barbera
Supervising Product Manager: Betsy Gentzler
Editorial Assistant: Jacalyn Clay
Design Coordinator: Holly Reid McLaughlin
Illustration Coordinator: Brett MacNaughton
Manufacturing Coordinator: Karin Duffield
Prepress Vendor: SPi Global

8th Edition

Printed in China

Library of Congress Cataloging-in-Publication Data
Alfaro-LeFevre, Rosalinda.
   Applying nursing process : the foundation for clinical reasoning / Rosalinda Alfaro-LeFevre. -- 8th ed.
      p. ; cm.
   Includes bibliographical references and index.
   ISBN 978-1-60913-697-0
   I. Title.
   [DNLM: 1. Nursing Process. WY 100]
   610.73--dc23

                                                                                    2012021976

About the Author

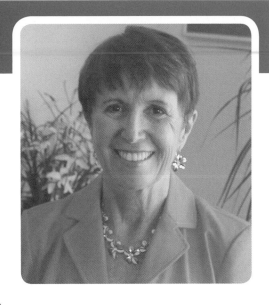

Known for making difficult content easy to understand, Rosalinda Alfaro-Lefevre, RN, MSN, ANEF is an energetic presenter and an AJN Book of the Year and a Sigma Theta Tau Best Pick award recipient. She is a National League for Nursing Academy of Nursing Education Fellow. Rosalinda immigrated to the United States from Argentina via Canada at the age of 10, and is well known nationally and internationally. Her work is available in seven languages. She has more than 20 years of clinical experience (mostly in ICU, CCU, and ED) and has taught in associate degree and baccalaureate nursing programs. She currently is the president of Teaching Smart/Learning Easy in Stuart, Florida, a company dedicated to helping people to acquire the intellectual and interpersonal skills needed to deal with today's personal and workplace challenges. You can learn more about Rosalinda at www.AlfaroTeachSmart.com.

Rosalinda Alfaro-LeFevre, RN, MSN, ANEF
President
Teaching Smart/Learning Easy
Stuart, Florida
www.AlfaroTeachSmart.com

To nurses everywhere and to generations past and future.... blessings in my life!

Louise Kelley Rochester (Dec 31, 1925 to Jan 30, 2010). Louise taught me how to bridge the generation gap before it was popular to do so. I wrote several editions of this book at her home in Duxbury, Massachusetts. (Courtesy of the Pape Family)

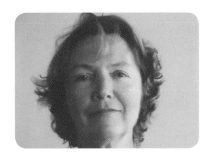

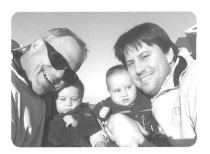

Jim, Reid, Grant, and Alex LeFevre, Kitty Hawk, North Carolina, 2011. (Courtesy of the LeFevre Family)

Alex, Reid, Grant, and Hillary LeFevre, New Bern, North Carolina, 2011. (Courtesy of the LeFevre Family)

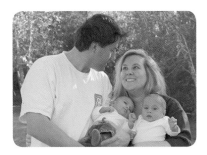

A NOTE OF THANKS

Without the timely and insightful reviews and advice of the experts listed on these pages, this book would not have been possible. The author also wishes to acknowledge the diligent work of the translators of this and previous editions.

USA

Ledjie Ballard, CRNA, MSN
Kalispell, Montana

Carol Bashford, RN, MSN, ACNS-BC, APRN
Associate Professor, Nursing
Miami University
Hamilton, Ohio

Deanne A. Blach, RN, MSN
Nurse Educator
DB Productions
Green Forest, Arkansas

Hilda Brito, RN-BC, MSN
Director of Special Programs/Staff Development
UHealth Bascom Palmer Eye Institute/ABLEH
Miami, Florida

Lori A. Brown, RN, MSN, CCRN
Lecturer
Department of Nursing
Gonzaga University
Spokane, Washington

Bonnie Carmack, MN, ARNP
Adjunct Faculty
Seminole State College Oviedo Campus
Oviedo, Florida

Charlotte Connerton, RN, MSN, FCN, CNE
Assistant Professor
Lakeview College of Nursing
Danville, Illinois

Janice Eilerman, RN, MSN
Course Coordinator/Instructor
James A. Rhodes State College
Lima, Ohio

Tracy S. Estes, RN, PhD, FNP-BC
Assistant Professor
School of Nursing
Virginia Commonwealth University
Richmond, Virginia

Rebecca S. Frugé, RN, PhD
Director, Graduate Nursing Program
Universidad Metropolitana
San Juan, Puerto Rico

Elizabeth E. Hand, RN, MS
Acute Care Education Specialist
Hands-on Nursing, PLLC
Tulsa, Oklahoma

Ruth Hansten, PhD, FACHE, MBA, BSN
Principle
Hansten Healthcare
Port Ludlow, Washington

Cheryl Herndon, ARNP, CNM, MSN
Director Aesthetic Services
Women's Health Specialists,
Jensen Beach, Florida

Cecelia E. Isales, RN, MSN
Assistant Nursing Professor
Carroll Community College
Westminster, Maryland

Sharon E. Johnson, MSN, RNC, NE-BC
Director, Home Health and Hospice
The Home Care Network
Main Line Health
Thomas Jefferson University Hospitals
Wayne, Pennsylvania

Nancy Konzelmann, MS, RN-BC, CPHQ
Nursing Professional Development Specialist
Port St. Lucie, Florida

Heidi Pape Laird
Systems Designer
Partners HealthCare
Boston, Massachusetts

Barbara Gillman Lamping, RN, MSN, MEd
Instructor
Good Samaritan College of Nursing and Health
    Sciences
Cincinnati, Ohio

Martha B. Lyman, RN, MSN, MPH
Nurse Navigator/Coordinator
Bryn Mawr Breast Center
Bryn Mawr, Pennsylvania

Jacquelyn P. Mayer, RN, MS
Associate Professor in Nursing
Good Samaritan College of Nursing and Health
    Sciences
Cincinnati, Ohio

Melani McGuire, RN, BSN
Staff Nurse, Emergency Department
Paoli Hospital
Paoli, Pennsylvania

Judith C. Miller, RN, MS
Nursing Tutorial & Consulting Services
Henniker, New Hampshire

Claudia Mitchell, RN, MSN
Associate Director UC BSN Program
University of Cincinnati–Clermont Campus
Batavia, Ohio

Jan Nash, RN, PhD, MSN, NEA-BC
Vice President/CNO Patient Services
Paoli Hospital
Paoli, Pennsylvania

Rochelle Nelson, RN, MS
Assistant Clinical Professor
College of Nursing
University of Wisconsin—Milwaukee
Milwaukee, Wisconsin

Cynthia O'Neal, RN, PhD
Assistant Professor
Texas Tech University Health Sciences Center
Lubbock, Texas

Terri Patterson, RN, MSN, CRRN, FIALCP
President
Nursing Consultation Services Ltd.
Plymouth Meeting, Pennsylvania

Catherine Pearsall, PhD, FNP, CNE
Associate Professor
St. Joseph's College
Patchogue, New York

William F. Perry, RN, MA
Informatics Consultant
Creekspace Informatics
Beavercreek, Ohio

Loretta Quigley, RN, MS
Associate Dean
St. Joseph's College
Syracuse, New York

Wendy Robinson, RN, PhD, FNP-BC
Vice President for Academic Affairs
Helene Fuld College of Nursing
New York, New York

Rose O Sherman, RN, EdD, NEA-BC, CNL, FAAN
Director, Nursing Leadership Institute
Associate Professor
Christine E. Lynn College of Nursing
Florida Atlantic University
Boca Raton, Florida

Carol R. Taylor, RN, PhD, MSN
Professor of Nursing and Medicine
Georgetown University
Washington, DC

Brent W. Thompson, RN, PhD
Associate Professor, Department of Nursing
West Chester University of Pennsylvania
West Chester, Pennsylvania

Elizabeth M. Tsarnas, ARNP, BC
Clinical Director
Volunteers in Medicine Clinic
Stuart, Florida

Theresa M. Valiga, RN, EdD, ANEF, FAAN
Professor & Director
Institute for Educational Excellence
Duke University School of Nursing
Durham, North Carolina

Diana White, RN, MS
Assistant Professor
School of Nursing and Allied Health
Tuskegee University
Tuskegee, Alabama

INTERNATIONAL

Miriam de Abreu Almeida, RN, PhD
Professor, School of Nursing
Universidade Federal do Rio Grande do Sul
Porto Alegre, Brazil

Dr. Judy Boychuk Duchscher, RN, PhD, MN, BScN
Assistant Professor—Faculty of Nursing
University of Calgary
Calgary, Alberta, Canada

Aiko Emoto
Professor Emeritus
Saniku Gakuin College
Chiba, Japan

Maria Teresa Luis, RN
Professor Emeritus
School of Nursing
University of Barcelona
Barcelona, Spain

Jeanne Michel, RN, PhD
Adjunct Professor, School of Nursing
Federal University of São Paulo
São Paulo, Brazil

Joanne Profetto-McGrath, RN, PhD
Professor and Vice Dean
Faculty of Nursing
University of Alberta
Edmonton, Alberta, Canada

I want to thank my husband, Jim, for his love, support, and sense of humor and fun and the rest of my family for being behind me all the way.

I also want to thank the following people for their belief in me and their contribution to my personal and professional growth: Louise and Nat Rochester, Heidi Laird, Terri Patterson, Ledjie Ballard, Annette Sophocles, Maria Sophocles, Melani McGuire, Carol Taylor, Patti Cleary, Terry Valiga, Ruth Hansten, Barbara Cohen, Mary Anne Rizzolo, Lynda Carpenito, Mary Jo Boyer, John Payne, Charlie and Nancy Lindsay, Becky Resh, Diane Verity, Nancy Flynn, Lorraine Locasale, Frank and Grace Nola, Chuck and Pat Morgan, Dan Hankison, Karen Smith, the past and present nurses at Paoli Hospital, and the faculty of the Villanova College of Nursing.

My special thanks go to the Nursing Education Editorial division of Lippincott Williams & Wilkins, especially to Patrick Barbera, Acquisitions Editor; Betsy Gentzler, Supervising Product Manager; and Jacalyn Clay, Editorial Assistant. I am indebted to Karen Ettinger of O'Donnell & Associates who coached me through an ambitious schedule and stayed on task to make the project manageable. Finally, I want to thank the sales and marketing department whose efforts have helped make this book a bestseller.

NURSING PROCESS: OUT OF THE BOX AND INTO EVIDENCE-BASED PRACTICE AND THE INFORMATION AGE

Staying true to my goal of applying nursing process in ways that are relevant to the sweeping changes we have in health care, this edition has been completely revised to address nurses' increased responsibilities related to both independent and multidisciplinary care. Nurses require highly developed critical thinking and clinical reasoning skills. Yet, many of them are confused about the relationship between nursing process and these two types of thinking. This book helps you understand these relationships and gives strategies and tools to help you develop the skills needed to thrive in our complex, challenging health care setting.

Use of the nursing process—*assess, diagnose, plan, implement,* and *evaluate*—is required by national practice standards, tested on the National Council Licensure Examination (NCLEX®), and forms the foundation for clinical reasoning. It underpins virtually all care models as an organizing framework and should resonate at the point of care. For example, skip the principles of *assessment* and *diagnosis* and it's easy to jump to conclusions, miss risks, and give care based on assumptions rather than evidence. Assessment errors and omissions are a major cause of adverse outcomes. If you fail to *plan* before *implementation,* the risk of adverse outcomes also increases. Skip *evaluation,* and reflective practice (not to mention patient safety) goes out the door. Because principles of nursing process are the building blocks for all care models, the nursing process is the first model nurses need to learn to "think like a nurse."

WHO SHOULD READ THIS BOOK?

If you need to do any of the following, this book is for you.

1. If you're a student and want to:
   - Gain the skills to think your way through NCLEX®.
   - Be more confident and competent in new clinical situations.
   - Set priorities to promote safety, efficiency, and patient-centered care.
2. If you're an educator or leader and need:
   - Everyone to be "on the same page," with clarity about the relationships among nursing process, critical thinking, and clinical reasoning
   - To prepare for Magnet status recognition by the American Nurses Credentialing Center (ANCC)
   - To prioritize learning to help students and nurses learn more efficiently

PRIORITIZING WHAT YOU TEACH

The biggest challenge for me to address came in Chapter 3, where we discuss how the use of nursing diagnosis is changing. I remain a strong believer in the benefits of learning the concept of nursing diagnosis—the idea that human responses are major nursing concerns and that nurses must identify problems related to how patients' lives are *impacted* by health issues and life changes. But, there are at least four main issues we need to address:

1. Increased emphasis on multidisciplinary care, evidence-based practice, and use of electronic health records is changing the terminology that's used. For example, on a multidisciplinary problem list or on NCLEX, you won't find terms like, *deficient knowledge, deficient fluid volume,* or *decreased intracranial adaptive capacity.* Rather, you'll find the well studied and commonly understood terms, *patient education, dehydration,* and *increased intracranial pressure.*
2. As nurses' accountability increases, they must be able to answer the question, "What are my independent responsibilities related to my patient's health issues (both medical and nursing problems)?" Answers to these questions arise from knowledge of qualifications and scope of practice in each particular setting.
3. Nurses' roles in surveillance and preventing complications must be taught early in their education. Much of the nursing care given today is aimed at managing clusters of *risk factors* that contribute to many different problems.
4. We must prioritize what we teach, and nurses must prioritize what they do. To avoid student overload and keep patients safe, we must teach the priority (most common and important) nursing issues *first.*

To help nurses learn the diagnostic process, I suggest the "working backwards" approach: Give beginners a list of the priority nursing issues (e.g., Box 3.3) and have them assess every patient for those concerns over and over again until they become priorities in their heads. As students and nurses move to various specialty units, the list should be adapted.

WHAT'S NEW TO THIS EDITION?

You get new information on:

- Developing Quality and Safety Education for Nurses (QSEN) competencies and Institute of Medicine (IOM) competencies
- Nurses' increased responsibilities related to medical, nursing, and other patient issues—making decisions about scope of practice
- How to set priorities and coordinate and delegate care safely and effectively
- Problem and risk identification—predicting and managing complications
- How terminology is changing to facilitate electronic records and improve communication among care providers

- Recognizing human responses and promoting independence and well-being
- Evidence-based practice, promoting patient-centered care, promoting health, ensuring surveillance, preventing errors, and activating the chain of command
- Creating healthy workplaces and safety and learning cultures that improve care and support and attract and retain good nurses
- Agreeing to a code of conduct that promotes ethical commitments to patients, organizations, and one another
- Patient-centered care—promoting partnerships and shared decision making
- The importance of thinking *with* electronic documentation and health information technology (rather than assuming these systems think *for* you)
- Quick priority assessments (QPA) to identify and prevent major patient problems *early*
- Using "Read Back" and "Repeat Back" rules to reduce communication errors
- Using structured tools such as the SBAR approach to improve hand-off communication
- The impact of chronic diseases and disabilities on people's lives
- The implications of moving from the *Diagnose and Treat* (DT) approach to the more proactive *Predict, Prevent, Manage, and Promote* (PPMP) approach
- Updated evidenced-based Critical Thinking Indicators—behaviors that promote critical thinking and clinical reasoning
- Using the 4-Circle CT Model to promote critical thinking
- Mapping to determine relationships and better understand patient issues
- The impact of real and simulated experiences on promoting reasoning and communication skills
- How thinking ahead, thinking-in-action, and thinking back (reflecting on thinking) improves clinical reasoning
- What to expect on NCLEX in relation to each phase of the nursing process
- New rules, tools, and strategies highlighted throughout

WHAT'S THE SAME?

To ensure a sound approach that's based on current standards, each chapter has been evaluated against requirements addressed in *Nursing Scope and Standards of Performance and Standards of Clinical Practice.*[1] Brain-based learning principles—strategies that help you get your brain "plugged in" to learning mode—are used throughout.

You also get:

- Lots of examples to make content relevant and easy to understand—the goal continues to be to give you a concise, engaging, user-friendly book
- A "big-picture" summary of how to use the nursing process as a tool for critical thinking (page facing inside front cover)
- A list of common complications associated with medical diagnoses, treatments, or diagnostic modalities (inside back cover and facing page)

- **More on:**
  - Nurses' roles in homes, communities, and multidisciplinary practice
  - Ethical, legal, cultural, and spiritual implications
  - The impact of cost containment and insurance requirements
  - How nurses' roles as diagnosticians and case managers continue to evolve
  - How to use critical pathways and standard plans to promote critical thinking
  - The importance of acquiring communication, interpersonal, and technical skills to promote critical thinking

FEATURES THAT HELP YOU LEARN

Great pains have been taken to make this a user-friendly book that helps you to move around the text as you please. The following elements are used to facilitate learning:

- Learning Outcomes written at the cognitive level of analysis precede each chapter.
- "What's in this chapter?" precedes content.
- A glossary at the end of the book defines key terms; difficult terms are clarified in the text by definition, discussion, and use within context.
- Illustrations are placed throughout to establish relationships and clarify text.
- Analogies, examples, and case studies are used to clarify information and demonstrate relevance of content.
- Rationales are highlighted as needed throughout the text.
- Questioning at the analysis level is used:
  1. During content presentation to stimulate curiosity and give clues to what's important
  2. After the content (in Critical Thinking and Clinical Reasoning Exercises) to reinforce key points and provide the opportunity to test and refine knowledge
- Content is presented in such a way that those who need structure have it, without restricting those who require more creative freedom.
- Key Points are given at the end of each chapter.

Other content and features retained from the previous editions include the following:

- **ANA Standards Related to This Chapter** are presented in chapter openers.
- **Rules**, given throughout the chapters, highlight important concepts.
- **Critical Thinking and Clinical Reasoning Exercises** are highlighted throughout to help you review and apply knowledge. (Example responses are provided at the end of the book.)
- **Try This on Your Own** exercises encourage you to learn more deeply through application and meaningful learning. These exercises don't have example responses at the end of the book because they're very individualized and would be too lengthy to cover.
- **Think About It** entries give "food for thought" to stimulate thinking and reinforce content.

- **Voices** excerpts offer quotations from nurses that are inspirational or exemplary of best practices.
- **This Chapter and NCLEX**, at the end of each chapter, lists important concepts and tips for applying chapter content during NCLEX.

A WORD ABOUT "PATIENT/CLIENT," "HE/SHE," AND STAKEHOLDER

Whenever possible, I use a fictitious name or "someone," "person," "consumer," or "individual" instead of "client" or "patient" to help us keep in mind that each client or patient is an individual who has unique needs, values, perceptions, and motivations. "He" and "she" are used interchangeably to avoid the awkwardness of using "he/she" over and over. The term *stakeholder* is used when describing *all* the people who are impacted by how care is given and what outcomes are achieved (e.g., patients, families, care providers, and insurance companies).

TEACHING AND LEARNING TOOLS

To facilitate mastery of this text's content, a teaching and learning package has been developed to assist faculty and students.

Instructor Resources

Tools to assist you with teaching your course are available upon adoption of this text on thePoint at http://thePoint.lww.com/Alfaro8e.

- **PowerPoint Presentations** for each chapter provide an easy way to integrate the textbook with the classroom. Presentations include multiple-choice and true/false questions to promote class participation.
- **Case Studies,** including three unfolding scenarios with questions (and suggested answers) for each chapter, provide an opportunity for students to apply their knowledge to a patient case similar to one they might encounter in practice.
- **Additional Handouts and Tools** to reinforce content are available for download from the author's Web site at www.AlfaroTeachSmart.com. These tools are free for personal use. If you require your students to purchase this text, you get unlimited use of these tools for educational purposes.

In addition, you'll receive Strategies for Effective Teaching and have access to all student resources described below.

Student Resources

Students can access free resources on thePoint using the codes printed in the front of their textbooks. Visit http://thePoint.lww.com/activate. Resources include the following:

- Free E-Book
- Expected Learning Outcomes
- Spanish–English Audio Glossary
- Nursing Professional Roles and Responsibilities

COMMENTS AND SUGGESTIONS WELCOMED

I welcome suggestions for improvement. Often the most significant changes are made based on student and faculty suggestions.

Rosalinda Alfaro-LeFevre, RN, MSN, ANEF
www.AlfaroTeachSmart.com

Reference

1. ANA. (2010). *Nursing scope and standards of performance and standards of clinical practice* (2nd ed.). Silver Springs, MD: nursesbooks.org.

Contents

Chapter 4   Planning   128

Chapter 5   Implementation   159

Chapter 6   Evaluation   188

Chapter 1

Overview of Nursing Process, Clinical Reasoning, and Nursing Practice Today

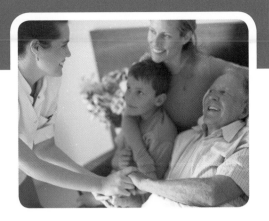

What's in This Chapter?

In this chapter, you get an overview of the nursing process and find out the answers to questions like, Why is the nursing process the foundation for clinical reasoning? What is the relationship between critical thinking and clinical reasoning? What do we have to know? What do we have to do first and why? You learn that there are five main reasons for studying the nursing process: (1) It's the first tool you need to learn to begin to "think like a nurse." (2) American Nurses Association (ANA) Standards mandate its use.[1] (3) It underpins virtually all care models and provides a tool for critical thinking and decision making. (4) It forms the foundation for National Council Licensure Examination (NCLEX®) and advanced certification exams. (5) Understanding nursing process *principles* is the key to practicing safely in today's computer-driven world. To help you apply what you learn from this chapter when you go to the clinical setting, you're introduced to key factors in today's health care that impact on your role as a nurse—including new information on national safety goals, your responsibilities related to activating the chain of command, and competencies that you must develop to be a safe and effective nurse. Stressing the importance of having good communication skills and knowing how to form partnerships with patients, families, and colleagues, this chapter helps you understand how to apply ethical principles to give outcome-focused, patient-centered care. Finally, you gain an understanding of *critical thinking indicators* (behaviors that promote critical thinking) and consider the importance of (1) developing critical thinking characteristics; (2) gaining theoretical and experiential knowledge; (3) acquiring interpersonal and technical skills; and (4) being willing and able to care.

Critical Thinking and Clinical Reasoning Exercises

Exercises 1.1   Nursing Process: The Foundation for Clinical Reasoning
Exercises 1.2   Developing Critical Thinking and Clinical Reasoning Skills

Expected Learning Outcomes

After studying this chapter, you should be able to:

1. Give three reasons why the nursing process is the foundation for clinical reasoning.
2. Describe how the terms critical thinking, clinical reasoning, nursing process, problem solving, and prevention are related.
3. Explain the relationships among the five phases of nursing process (*Assessment, Diagnosis, Planning, Implementation*, and *Evaluation*).
4. Give at least four benefits of using the nursing process.
5. Address how clinical reasoning is affected by standards, policies, ethics codes, and laws (individual state practice acts).
6. Explain why you need to understand nursing process *principles* to be able to safely use standard and electronic plans.
7. Name at least five trends in health care that impact on nurses' thinking.
8. Compare and contrast the nursing process and the process physicians use to treat medical problems.
9. Address why moving from a culture of blame to a culture of safety is needed to make keeping patients safe top priority.
10. Decide where you stand in relation to developing Quality and Safety Education for Nurses (QSEN) Competencies.
11. Activate the chain of command as indicated by patient conditions.
12. Explain the meaning of *"Assess, Re-assess, Revise, and Record"* and *"Think Ahead, Think-in-Action, and Think Back."*
13. Apply seven ethical principles and ANA Code of Ethics to planning and giving care.
14. Discuss how real and simulated experiences impact on your ability to develop clinical reasoning skills.
15. Explain how following a code of conduct promotes healthy workplaces and learning environments in context of a culture of safety.
16. Determine at least five Critical Thinking Indicators (CTIs) you want to develop or improve.
17. Use the 4-Circle CT Model to identify skills you need to develop.
18. Start to develop the communication and interpersonal skills needed for critical thinking.
19. Address what it takes to be willing and able to demonstrate caring behaviors.
20. Use the nursing process as a tool for clinical reasoning and critical thinking in clinical, classroom, and testing situations.

NURSING PROCESS: THE FOUNDATION FOR CLINICAL REASONING

Use of the nursing process—required by national practice standards and tested on the National Council Licensure Examination and other certification tests—is the foundation for clinical reasoning. It gives you an organized, systematic way of thinking about patient care. According to ANA standards, the nursing process is a critical thinking model used to promote a competent level of care, encompasses all significant actions taken by registered nurses, and forms the foundation for decision making.[1,2] For these reasons, the nursing process is the *first* model you need to learn to "think like a nurse."

Today, care is often driven by electronic health records (EHR) and decision-support systems. Yet, having nursing process principles *in your head* is the key to developing thinking habits that promote safe, effective care at the point of care (e.g., at the bedside). Developing these habits makes the difference between keeping patients safe and putting them in harm's way. It may also be your defense if ever accused of negligence. When courts examine whether standards of care have been met, they check patient records to determine if all phases of the nursing process—*Assessment, Diagnosis, Planning, Implementation*, and *Evaluation*—were recorded.

Applying nursing process principles helps you:

1. Organize and prioritize your patient care
2. Keep the focus on what's important—patient safety, health status, quality of life, and how the patient is responding to care
3. Form thinking habits that help you gain the confidence and skills you need to think to reason your way through clinical, theoretical, and testing situations
4. Use EHR and decision-support systems as they are meant to be used—as guides that boost your brain, not replace it

The nursing process is more than something that guides formal care planning and documentation. It's what must guide nurses' thinking on a daily basis. At every turn, you must be assessing, diagnosing, planning, implementing, and evaluating. Figure 1.1 maps the nursing process "in action." Notice that two of the boxes are shaded to stress the importance of assessing before, during, and after you give care.

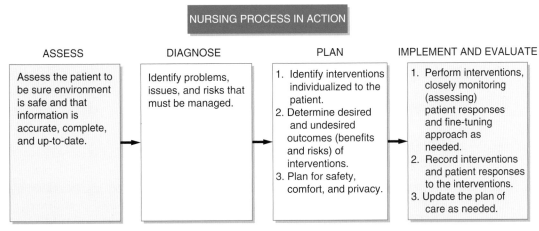

NURSING PROCESS IN ACTION

ASSESS	DIAGNOSE	PLAN	IMPLEMENT AND EVALUATE
Assess the patient to be sure environment is safe and that information is accurate, complete, and up-to-date.	Identify problems, issues, and risks that must be managed.	1. Identify interventions individualized to the patient. 2. Determine desired and undesired outcomes (benefits and risks) of interventions. 3. Plan for safety, comfort, and privacy.	1. Perform interventions, closely monitoring (assessing) patient responses and fine-tuning approach as needed. 2. Record interventions and patient responses to the interventions. 3. Update the plan of care as needed.

FIGURE 1.1   Nursing process in action. Two boxes are shaded because they both address the importance of assessment. (© 2011 R. Alfaro-LeFevre. www.AlfaroTeachSmart.com)

RULE   The nursing process consists of five phases—*Assessment, Diagnosis, Planning, Implementation*, and *Evaluation (ADPIE)*. Rather than being linear, with a beginning and end, the nursing process is a continuous cycle of phases. ANA standards address six standards, considering *Outcome Identification* separately after *Diagnosis*, and before *Planning*. NCLEX uses five phases, as we do in this book. We address *Outcome Identification* as a key part of *Planning*.

GOALS OF NURSING

An important starting point for learning about the nursing process is having a good understanding of the ultimate goals of nursing—what do we as nurses aim to do?

Think about the following main goals of nursing.

- Prevent illness and promote, maintain, or restore health (in terminal illness, the goal is a peaceful death)
- Maximize sense of well-being, independence, and ability to function in desired roles (as defined by the patient)
- Provide cost-effective, efficient care that pays attention to individual biological, social, spiritual, and cultural needs
- Continually work to improve patient outcomes, care practices, and consumer satisfaction

CRITICAL THINKING VERSUS CLINICAL REASONING

The terms *critical thinking* (CT) and *clinical reasoning* (CR) are often used interchangeably, as we do in this book. Many of the principles of CT and CR are the same. But, there is a slight difference between these terms. *Clinical reasoning* is a specific term that refers to the assessment and management of patient problems at the point of care—for example, applying nursing process at the bedside. For reasoning about other clinical issues such as promoting teamwork and streamlining work flow, nurses usually use the term *critical thinking*. Critical thinking is a *broad term* that includes clinical reasoning. Keep in mind the following points.

Critical Thinking and Clinical Reasoning are Outcome-Focused Thinking That[3]:

- **Is based on principles of nursing process, problem solving, and the scientific method** (requires forming opinions and making decisions based on evidence).
- **Is guided by standards, policies, ethics codes, and laws** (individual state practice acts and state boards of nursing).

- **Focuses on safety and quality,** constantly reevaluating, self-correcting, and striving to improve.
- **Carefully identifies the key problems, issues, and risks involved,** including patients, families, and key stakeholders in decision making early in the process. *Stakeholders* are the people who will be most affected (patients and families) or from whom requirements will be drawn (caregivers, insurance companies, third-party payers, health care organizations).
- **Is driven by patient, family, and community needs,** as well as nurses' needs to give competent efficient care (e.g., streamlining charting to free nurses for patient care).
- **Calls for strategies that make the most of human potential** and compensate for problems created by human nature (e.g., finding ways to prevent errors, using technology, and overcoming the powerful influence of personal views).

RULE Critical thinking is "important thinking" that has to happen to assess, prevent, or manage any situation. In nursing, this means using evidence-based strategies (strategies that research has shown to be effective) in all phases of the nursing process.

HOW THE NURSING PROCESS PROMOTES SAFE, EFFECTIVE REASONING

Consider how the following characteristics of nursing process promote safe, effective reasoning.

Purposeful, Organized, and Systematic. Each phase is designed to achieve a specific purpose. For example, *Assessment* aims to *gather* the facts you need to determine health status. *Diagnosis* aims to *analyze* those facts to identify the problems and risks involved. Because the phases guide you to think in a systematic, organized way, they help you to avoid missing anything important.

Humanistic. Based on the belief that we must consider patients' unique interests, values, needs, and culture, the nursing process guides you to focus holistically on the body, mind, and spirit. It pushes you to consider health problems *in context of how they impact on each person's sense of well-being and ability to be independent.* For instance, suppose "Bob" has severe arthritis. You work to understand how it impacts on his ability to work, to do desired activities, to sleep, and to function in his role as father of three young children.

Dynamic Cycle. While the phases progress one after the other, the nursing process is actually a dynamic cycle. For example, if things aren't going well during

Implementation, you go back to *Assessment*, to make sure you have the most correct, up-to-date data.

Proactive. The nursing process stresses the need to not only treat *problems* but also prevent them by managing risk factors and encouraging healthy behaviors, such as daily exercise and stress management.

Evidence-Based. It mandates that judgments, decisions, and actions be based on the best evidence. Strict documentation requirements ensure that we have the data we need to manage care and to help researchers study care practices and improve them.

Outcome-Focused and Cost-Effective. Applying nursing process principles helps you figure out how to achieve the best results (outcomes) in the most efficient and cost-effective way.

Intuitive and Logical. Principles of nursing process push you to acknowledge patterns and intuitive hunches, then to look for evidence that supports your intuition.

Reflective, Creative, and Improvement-Oriented. It stresses the need for ongoing evaluation, requiring us to continually reflect on patient responses (outcomes) and our process (how we give care), so that we can make corrections early. Creativity and continuous improvement of nursing care are also important. We must think creatively about how to improve both the process of giving care and the results (patient outcomes).

Recorded in a Standard Way. Recording all phases in precise ways improves communication, and prevents errors, omissions, and unnecessary repetitions. It also leaves a "paper or electronic trail" that later can be analyzed to evaluate patient care and do the studies needed to advance nursing and improve the health care quality and efficiency.

RULE **Using standard and electronic plans safely requires having nursing process principles *in your head*.** If you don't understand the purpose of each phase, the relationship among the phases, and how each step is accomplished, it's like using a calculator without ever having learned what it means to add, subtract, multiply, or divide. To be an independent thinker who's able to give safe, effective care and improve current practices, gain an understanding of the *reasoning* behind the nursing process.

NURSING PROCESS PHASES

Let's examine what you do during each nursing process phase and how the phases are related.

Five Phases

Here's a brief description of what you do during each phase of the nursing process:

1. **Assessment.** Collect and record all the information you need to:
   - Predict, detect, prevent, and manage actual and potential health problems
   - Promote optimum health, independence, and well-being
   - Clarify expected outcomes (results)
2. **Diagnosis.** Analyze the data you gathered, draw conclusions, and determine whether there are:
   - Risks for safety or infection transmission (deal with these immediately)
   - Signs or symptoms that need evaluation by a more qualified professional (report these immediately)
   - Actual and potential health problems requiring nursing or medical management
   - Risk factors requiring nursing or medical management
   - Issues that aren't quite clear, but require further investigation
   - Learning needs that must be addressed
   - Patient resources, strengths, and use of healthy behaviors
   - Health states that are satisfactory but could be improved

RULE   **Unless you're an Advanced Practice Nurse (APN), state laws prohibit you from making medical diagnoses independently.**[4] You are, however, accountable for giving high priority to assessing and reporting signs and symptoms that may indicate the need for attention from a professional more qualified than you. For example, if your patient has signs and symptoms of a myocardial infarction (e.g., chest pain and shortness of breath), you're accountable for: (1) suspecting that this could be the problem; (2) recognizing that it is a high priority; (3) doing what you can to address the problem (e.g., raise the head of the bed); and (4) reporting it immediately. This is called "Activating the Chain of Command" (follow policies and procedures for getting help; be persistent—stay with the problems until your patients get the qualified help they need).

3. **Planning.** Clarify expected outcomes (results), set priorities, and determine interventions (nursing actions). The interventions are designed to:
   - Detect, prevent, and manage health problems and risk factors
   - Promote optimum function, independence, and sense of well-being
   - Achieve the expected outcomes safely and efficiently
4. **Implementation.** Put the plan into action:
   - Assess the patient to determine current status—decide whether the patient is ready and the interventions are still appropriate.
   - Perform the interventions (nursing actions).
   - Reassess the patient to determine end results (outcomes).
   - Make immediate changes as needed.
   - Chart nursing actions and patient responses.

RULE Remember "Assess, Re-assess, Revise, Record." *Assess* patients before you perform nursing actions. *Re-assess* them to determine their responses immediately *after* you perform nursing actions. *Revise* your approach if needed. *Record* patient responses and any changes you made in the plan.

5. **Evaluation.** Do a comprehensive patient assessment to decide whether expected outcomes have been met or whether new problems have emerged.
   ● Decide whether to modify or terminate the plan.
   ● Plan for ongoing continuous assessment and improvement.

RULE When you're a novice or in unfamiliar situations, use the nursing process in a strict step-by-step way to be sure that you don't miss anything important. When you are in familiar situations—after the phases are like second nature—you'll use the nursing process in dynamic ways. For example, experienced ICU nurses can take one look at their patients and know that something's wrong. Their eyes flash to the monitor—checking heart rate and rhythm. They may jump to the *Intervention* phase, raising or lowering the head of the bed depending on instincts, before completing *Diagnosis*. At same time, they talk with the patient and grab a blood pressure cuff to continue *Assessment*.

Table 1.1 compares the Nursing Process and the Problem-Solving Method. Notice how the problem-solving method begins when you encounter a problem. The proactive nursing process stresses the need for continuous assessment for risk factors (even when no problems exist).

Table 1.1 Nursing Process Versus Problem-Solving Method

Nursing Process	Problem-Solving Method
Assessment: Continuously collecting data about health status to monitor for evidence of health problems and risk factors that may contribute to health problems (e.g., smoking).	**Encountering a problem:** Collecting data about the problem.
Diagnosis: Analyzing data to identify actual and potential health problems, risk factors, and strengths.	**Analyzing data** to determine exactly what the problem is.
Planning: Determining desired outcomes (benefits expected to be seen in the patient after care is done) and identifying interventions to achieve the outcomes.	**Making a plan** of action.
Implementation: Putting the plan into action and observing initial responses.	**Putting the plan into action.**
Evaluation: Determining how well the outcomes have been met and deciding whether changes need to be made. Looking for ways to make things better.	**Evaluating the results.**

NOTE: Throughout this book, the term *medical problem* refers to diseases or trauma diagnosed by primary care providers such as physicians or advanced practice nurses. The term *medical order* refers to interventions and treatments prescribed by primary care providers. The terms used to describe specific conditions throughout are the most common, evidence-based terms, rather than terms belonging to any specific taxonomy. For example, *dehydration* (a well studied problem) is used rather than *fluid volume deficit.*

Relationships Among the Phases

The nursing process phases are fluid, and interrelated, as described in the following section.

Assessment and Diagnosis

The following shows *Assessment* and *Diagnosis* as phases that overlap.

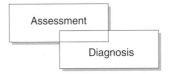

***Assessment* and *Diagnosis* are closely related and overlap for two reasons**:

1. Accurate diagnosis depends on accurate and complete assessment.
2. As you gather information during *Assessment*, you start to analyze and interpret what it means before you have a complete "diagnostic picture." For example: You are interviewing Mrs. King as part of a preadmission assessment for surgery. You notice a rash on her arms and legs and make a tentative diagnosis (Mrs. King may have some sort of skin or allergy problem) as you focus your assessment to get more information.

Diagnosis and Planning

The following shows *Diagnosis* and *Planning* overlapping.

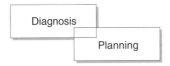

Diagnosis **and** *Planning* **are related for several reasons:**

1. Accurate planning depends on accurate diagnosis. If you miss problems or misunderstand them, you waste time developing a plan to solve the wrong problems. The real problems may go undetected and become worse due to neglect or incorrect treatment.

2. To achieve the overall desired outcome of care—that is, that the person is able to be as independent as possible—you must develop specific outcomes for each problem or diagnosis that must be managed to stay on track for expected discharge. For example, if *constipation* is a major problem, one outcome might be the person has a soft bowel movement at least every other day.

3. The interventions you identify during *Planning* must be designed to prevent, resolve, or manage the problems identified during *Diagnosis*. For example, for *constipation*, you plan interventions to promote bowel regularity (e.g., teaching the need for adequate hydration, dietary roughage, and so forth).

4. There are times when you have to act quickly, implementing a plan of action, before you identify all the problems. For example, if you encounter life-threatening problems, take immediate action. After the situation is under control, complete the *Diagnosis* phase by analyzing all of the data in depth.

5. It's important to incorporate the resources and strengths you identify during *Diagnosis* into the plan. For example, if you learn that someone is unable to plan meals but has relatives who are willing to help, use the relatives as a resource (e.g., teaching relatives how to include high-roughage foods in the diet).

Planning and Implementation

The following diagram shows *Planning* and *Implementation* overlapping.

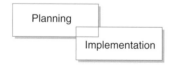

Planning **and** *Implementation* **are related and overlap for two main reasons:**

1. The plan guides interventions performed during *Implementation*.
2. As you implement the plan, you often need to fine-tune it to get the results you need. Sometimes, you even have to go back and check whether your assessment and diagnosis information is correct.

Implementation and Evaluation

The following shows *Implementation* and *Evaluation* overlapping.

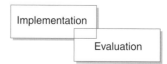

Implementation **and** *Evaluation* **overlap for an obvious reason:** *Evaluation* **is an important** *part* **of** *Implementation.* As you implement the plan, you evaluate your patients' responses carefully, and make changes early as needed.

Evaluation and the Other Phases

The following diagram shows the nursing process as a *cycle* that begins with *Assessment*, goes *on through the other phases to Evaluation*, and then back to *Assessment* (you assess the patient to determine current status and evaluate outcome achievement). The shading of the *Planning* and *Evaluation* boxes indicates the important relationship between *Evaluation* and *Planning:* Assuming that your diagnoses are accurate and your outcomes are appropriate, the ultimate question to be answered during *Evaluation* is, "Have we achieved the outcomes determined during *Planning?*"

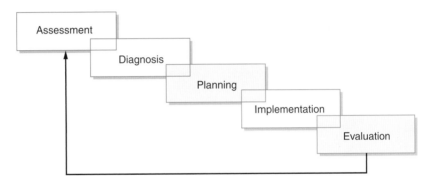

Comprehensive evaluation involves examining what happened in all of the other steps, as shown in the following diagram.

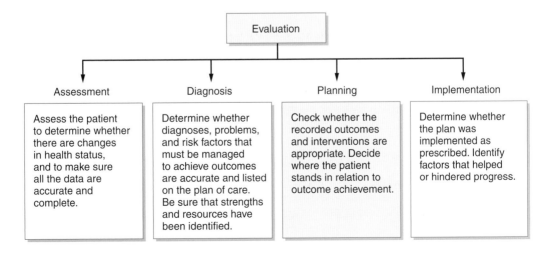

RULE When applying nursing process, remember the importance of thinking ahead, thinking in action, and thinking back (reflecting on the care given).[7] **Think ahead** (be proactive—anticipate what might happen and how you can be prepared). **Think in action** (pay attention to what's going on in your head as you "think on your feet," gathering and putting information together). **Think back** (reflect on your thinking to decide what you can learn from what happened, what influenced your thinking, and what you can do better next time—this usually requires chart review and journaling or dialoguing with others to make your thoughts explicit).

To increase your understanding of the nursing process, review the case scenario in Box 1.1.

Box 1.1   Case Scenario: Applying Nursing Process When Caring for an Elderly Man at Home

Assessment

Mr. Martin is 80 years old and lives alone. He wants to be independent and keeps a clean home. However, today he has a cold, is weak, and states that he is feeling very tired. Other than that, his health is unchanged.

Diagnosis

You analyze the above data and realize that Mr. Martin's age and fatigue put him at risk for falls. You recognize that his desire for independence is a strength, but you also know that it might be a weakness because he may not ask for help. You tell him that you'd like him to have some extra help while he's ill because you're concerned that his weakness puts him at risk for falls.

Planning

Together with Mr. Martin, you agree on the following outcome: Mr. Martin will be free of injury with reduced risk factors for falls. You then develop a plan to prevent falls (e.g., you arrange furniture so things are out of the way or easy to grasp for balance, you stress the importance of adequate nutrition and hydration with a cold, and you ask who might be able to come and help for a few days). You plan to monitor his blood pressure, because you know that low blood pressure is a risk factor for falls.

Implementation

You monitor him closely, checking vital signs, monitoring food and fluid intake, and finding out if he has help each day. Knowing of his desire for independence, you stress the importance of accepting help from others. You encourage him to keep up his strength by avoiding being in bed all day.

Evaluation

You assess Mr. Martin to determine whether he is free from injury and whether the risk factors for falls are still present. If he has regained his strength, encourage him to continue his usual independent lifestyle. If not, reassess his health status and decide whether to make changes in the plan.

BENEFITS OF USING THE NURSING PROCESS

The nursing process complements what other health care professionals do by focusing on both the medical problems and the *impact* of medical problems and treatment plans on patients' lives (human responses). For example, if someone has a broken leg, the physician focuses on treating the broken bones, and the physical therapist focuses on promoting muscle strength and balance. You, as the nurse, follow the medical treatment plan, but focus on the *whole person*—for example, how to manage pain holistically, whether there's a risk for injury or problem with skin integrity, and what inconveniences the patient has.

This holistic focus helps to ensure that interventions are tailored to the *individual*, not just the disease. Can you think what it would be like if you were hospitalized with a head laceration, a fractured arm, and a bruised kidney and everyone focused only on your medical problems? Can you imagine lying there with daily visits from a surgeon to check your head, an orthopedist to look at your arm, a urologist to check your kidney, and no one there to be concerned with how *you* are doing—to ask about you (what things would help you be more independent and comfortable)?

Consider the following example of the difference between how a physician and a nurse might analyze the same patient's data.

EXAMPLE

Physician's data (disease focus): "Mrs. Garcia has pain and swelling in all joints. Diagnostic studies indicate that she has rheumatoid arthritis. We will start her on a course of anti-inflammatory drugs to treat the rheumatoid arthritis." (Focus is on treating the arthritis.)

Nurse's data (holistic focus, considering the diseases, the patient's human response to the diseases, and how the diseases impact on the person's ability to function independently): "Mrs. Garcia has pain and swelling in all joints, making it difficult for her to feed and dress herself. She has voiced that it's difficult to feel worthwhile when she can't even feed herself. She states that she is depressed because she misses seeing her two small grandchildren. We need to develop a plan to help her with her pain, to assist her with feeding and dressing, to work through feelings of low self-esteem, and for special visitations with the grandchildren." (Focus is on Mrs. Garcia.)

Table 1.2 compares the nursing process and the medical process.

NURSING PROCESS IN CONTEXT OF TODAY'S CLINICAL SETTING

To help you know what to expect when applying nursing process in the clinical setting, this section summarizes key issues and trends that affect patient care today. For example, in the past, we were very involved with developing plans "from scratch." Today, in many cases we *adapt* standard plans already developed for specific

Table 1.2   Comparison of Nursing and Medical Process

Nursing Process	Medical Process
Focuses on body, mind, and spirit and aims to maximize health and independence.	Focuses on treating diseases, pathophysiology, and trauma.
Mainly considers how peoples' lives are *affected by* problems with organ and system function (human responses).	Mainly considers problems with organ and system function.
Manages medical problems under physician's orders or protocols. Prevents medical problems through proactive nursing care.	Manages medical problems independently. Delegates some treatments to nurses.

conditions. To reflect these changes, throughout this book, we'll approach using the nursing process from two perspectives:

1. How to create a comprehensive plan of care from beginning to end, applying the steps of *Assessment, Diagnosis, Planning, Implementation, and Evaluation.* Studying each of the phases in depth will help you gain insights needed to be able to move on to using the nursing process in dynamic ways.
2. How to adapt existing plans to make them appropriate for each unique individual.

Let's begin this section on today's clinical setting by examining the importance of making patient safety the number one concern of all health care providers.

Patient Safety and Welfare Is Top Priority

After a report by the Institute of Medicine (IOM), *To Err Is Human,*[5] stated that medical errors contributed to almost 100,000 deaths in the United States every year, patient safety and welfare has become top priority. Safety organizations stress that to reduce errors, we need to change "cultures of blame" to "cultures of safety." In a culture of blame, those who make mistakes are personally blamed and punitive actions are taken against them. In a culture of safety, the emphasis is on identifying *all the contributing factors*. We examine errors carefully to determine the root (main) causes. For example, the root cause of medication errors may not be knowledge errors, but system failures, such as look-alike drugs being stored side by side. Other examples of system problems that contribute to mistakes include lack of IV pumps to prevent rapid infusion, nurses who are overworked or placed in positions that require knowledge and skills beyond their capabilities, and inconvenient hand sanitation stations. In a culture of safety, when errors happen, a root-cause analysis is done to study both the individual's role *and* the system's role in the mistake. Only then can we identify comprehensive strategies and procedures to prevent future errors.

RULE   **Keep patients safe—move from a "culture of blame"** (where workers hide mistakes due to fear of punitive actions) **to a "culture of safety"** (where high priority is given to reporting mistakes, identifying systems that are error-prone, and working together to develop systems that keep patients safe).

The following shows examples of national safety goals:

1. Eliminate wrong-site, wrong-patient, and wrong-procedure surgery.
2. Reduce infections through improved hand washing, use of user-friendly protective barriers, and universal precautions.
3. Improve the:
   - Accuracy of patient identification
   - Effectiveness of communication among caregivers
   - Safety of using high-alert medications and IV pumps
   - Effectiveness of clinical alarm systems

For up-to-date Patient Safety Goals, enter "Patient Safety" in the search field at www.jointcommission.org.

Quality and Safety Education for Nurses Competencies

In response to the IOM's position that all health care providers must be able to provide patient-centered care, work in interdisciplinary teams, and employ evidence-based practice (EBP), quality improvement, and informatics (use computers to manage and process information), nurse educators developed the QSEN project (www.qsen.org). The QSEN goal is to prepare nurses to gain the knowledge, skills, and attitudes needed to continuously improve the quality and safety of the health care systems.[6] QSEN stresses the need for all nurses to develop the following competencies, quoted from www.qsen.org.

QSEN Competencies

- **Patient-Centered Care:** Recognize the patient or designee as the source of control and full partner in providing compassionate and coordinated care based on respect for the patient's preferences, values, and needs.
- **Teamwork and Collaboration:** Function effectively within nursing and interprofessional teams, fostering open communication, mutual respect, and shared decision making to achieve quality patient care.
- **Evidence-Based Practice:** Integrate best current evidence with clinical expertise and patient/family preferences and values for delivery of optimal health care.
- **Quality Improvement (QI):** Use data to monitor the outcomes of care processes and use improvement methods to design and test changes to continuously improve the quality and safety of health care systems.
- **Safety:** Minimize risk of harm to patients and providers through both system effectiveness and individual performance.

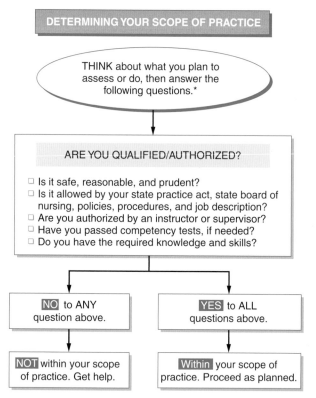

FIGURE 1.2   Scope of practice and decision making. Scope of practice varies from state to state, depending on state practice acts and State Board of Nursing (SBN) rules and regulations. When in doubt, ask your clinical educator or supervisor. You can also find out contact information for your SBN at https://www.ncsbn.org/nclex.htm. To review a model nursing practice act, go to https://www.ncsbn.org/2886.htm?iframe=true&width=500&height=270

Legal and Scope of Practice Concerns

One of the most challenging questions for beginning nurses is, What am I legally authorized to do? Your scope of practice—what you're legally allowed to assess or do—is defined by individual state practice acts and state boards of nursing. It varies depending on your qualifications and organizational policies. To keep patients safe and help you avoid overstepping your boundaries, study Figure 1.2, which gives a guide to help you make these types of decisions.

Giving Ethical Patient-Centered Care

To advocate for your patients and give ethical care, you need to have a good under-standing of the following principles.

Seven Ethical Principles

Autonomy. People have the right to make decisions based on (1) their own values and beliefs, (2) adequate information given free from coercion, and (3) sound reasoning that considers all alternatives

Beneficence. Aim to do good and avoid harm.

Justice. Treat people fairly; aim for equality.

Fidelity. Keep promises and don't make promises you can't keep.

Veracity. Tell the truth. Be honest with patients, families, and peers.

Accountability. Take responsibility for the consequences of your actions.

Confidentiality. Keep information private (this is also law).

Following ANA Ethics Code

Think about your responsibilities in relation to the following key points, summarized from the ANA's *Code of Ethics for Nurses*[8]:
Choosing to be a nurse means making the commitment to:

- **Practice with compassion and respect for each person's dignity, worth, and unique individuality.** This applies to patients, families, and coworkers, regardless of the nature of their health problems, socioeconomic status, or culture. Understand that human beings have the right to self-determination—to make their own decisions based on adequate information and guided by their own values and beliefs.
- **Keep your primary commitment to consumers (patient, family, group, or community).** It's your responsibility to promote, advocate, and protect the health, safety, privacy, and rights of consumers. Recognize conflict of interests (when your own values and beliefs are at odds with those of patients' or other caregivers). Advocate in patients' best interest.
- **Maintain a professional relationship.** Although giving care is personal, often requiring a friendly attitude, maintain professional boundaries. You're the professional and patients aren't your friends.
- **Ensure safe, effective, efficient, ethical care by collaborating with others.** Get second opinions. Delegate tasks as needed. Involve patients and key caregivers to make decisions and establish shared goals. Recognize when you have an ethical dilemma that requires input from qualified ethicists. Get informed consent from patients involved in research studies.
- **Respect your own worth and dignity.** Incorporate healthy behaviors into your life. Strive to grow personally and professionally. Be responsible and accountable for your nursing practice (this includes your direct patient care and the overall accountability of the nursing profession). Broaden your knowledge and seek out

learning experiences. Help advance the profession by contributing to practice, education, administration, and knowledge development (this improves patient care and your own worth and employability).

● **Participate in establishing, maintaining, and improving the health care environment.** Advocate for work conditions that are conducive to providing quality health care.

● **Get involved in professional organizations.** Help articulate nursing values, shape policies, and maintain and improve the integrity of the profession and its practice.

RULE **Agreeing to a code of conduct** that focuses on patient safety and welfare first and promotes teamwork helps you establish ethical, trusting relationships with patients, families, and other health team members.

Additional Clinical Issues Impacting Reasoning

The following lists additional workplace issues impacting clinical reasoning.

Importance of Developing Healthy Work and Learning Environments Stressed. Nursing organizations recognize the importance of providing a climate that's respectful, healing, humane, and safe. For links for healthy workplace, violence and injury, prevention, and other topics, go to www.cdc.gov/.

Maintaining Privacy Is Law. Patient privacy is guarded by the Health Insurance Portability and Accountability Act (HIPAA) of 1996.

Diverse Responsibilities. Nurses at all levels—in hospitals, homes, skilled nursing facilities, nursing homes, and communities—are more accountable for diagnosis, prevention, and management of various health problems. Other responsibilities include primary health care, patient education, health promotion, rehabilitation, self-care, and alternative methods of healing. In many cases, nurses are responsible for overseeing care given by unlicensed workers.

Nursing Roles in Collaborative Practice Expand. Nurses increasingly diagnose and manage problems that once were in the medical domain, depending on competency (knowledge, skills, and credentials) and authority (what's allowed based on laws and facility policies). For example, in critical care units, nurses diagnose and treat hypertension, congestive heart failure, and numerous other problems using well-defined clinical protocols.

Monitoring Role (Nursing Surveillance) Stressed. The importance of having skilled nurses present to monitor signs and symptoms to detect, prevent, and treat potential complications early is stressed. Nurses are responsible for monitoring for—and reporting—unsafe practices that may lead to errors, safety problems, or infection transmission.

Teamwork is Cornerstone of Safe, Effective Care. Knowing how to be an effective team member—working collaboratively with doctors, pharmacists, nutritionists, physical therapists, respiratory therapists, and other nurses and workers enhances patient care, prevents mistakes, and shortens length of stays. Box 1.2 summarizes the diverse skills needed to work as an effective member of the health care team.

Box 1.2   **Diverse Skills Required to Be a Nurse Today***

You must be able to:

- **Be flexible and adapt** to different settings and circumstances, identifying new knowledge, skills, and perspectives needed to practice proficiently.
- **Solve problems, think critically and creatively,** and respond to clinical complexity.
- **Make independent and shared decisions,** considering costs and involving clients and their families as partners.
- **Meet deadlines,** demonstrating responsibility, self-esteem, self-confidence, self-management, sociability, and integrity.
- **Collaborate** with professionals, peers, patients, families, and other health care workers by cultivating communication, interpersonal, and group-thinking skills.
- **Think holistically,** looking after the entire patient, considering both disease process and the impact of the disease and associated problems on individual lifestyles.
- **Promote wellness** through education, health screening, reduction of risk factors, and control of symptoms and causative factors.
- **Make ethical decisions** based on ethical principles.
- **Teach and learn efficiently** by taking advantage of individual learning style preferences.
- **Assess and respond to the diverse needs** and values of various groups (e.g., various cultures, age groups, and those of different sexual orientation).
- **Advocate for clients, families, and nurses** with the ability to present a case and listen to needs of others and a commitment to promote access to health care for all people, regardless of ability to pay.
- **Lead, supervise, and listen to and grasp** the needs of followers.
- **Manage information,** and organize and maintain files using computers to assist in interpretation and processing of information.
- **Use technology:** select equipment and tools, maintain and troubleshoot equipment, apply technology to tasks, and evaluate the appropriateness of complex and costly equipment.
- **Use resources: allocate time, money, materials, space, and human resources** in the development of programs and delivery of care.
- **Assess social and organizational systems;** monitor and correct performance; design or improve systems.
- **Determine the role of community services** in health care delivery, providing support as needed.
- **Provide customer service** with a clear understanding of what's important to consumers.

*List compiled from many documents on 21st century skills.

Stakeholders Included in Decisions. We know the importance of including key stakeholders—those who are most affected by the plan of care, for example, patients, families, caregivers, and third-party payers—early in the planning process.

Partnerships Nurtured. To ensure common goals, the importance of developing partnerships is stressed. Examples of key partnerships today are doctor–nurse, teacher–learner, and nurse–patient partnerships. Patients are encouraged to speak up and take an active role in all nursing care (see Box 1.3).

Meeting Diverse Patient Needs (Population-Based Care). Nurses must be able to meet the needs of diverse populations (patients of certain cultures, religions, age groups, languages, or sexual orientation). For more information, download the following documents:
- *Advancing Effective Communication, Cultural Competence and Patient- and Family-Centered Care: A Road Map for Hospitals*, available at http://www.jointcommission.org/Advancing_Effective_Communication/
- Detailed brochures on Patients' Rights in English and Spanish from http://www.jointcommission.org/Speak_Up__Know_Your_Rights/

Box 1.3	**Improve Safety: Urge Your Patients To Speak Up®**

Encourage your patients to be active, involved, and informed participants on the health care team. Tell them that the following simple steps are based on research which shows that patients who take part in making decisions about their health care are more likely to have better outcomes.

Speak up if you have questions or concerns, and if you don't understand, ask again. It's your body and you have a right to know.

Pay attention to the care you are receiving. Make sure you're getting the right treatments and medications by the right health care professionals. Don't assume anything.

Educate yourself about your diagnosis, the medical tests you are undergoing, and your treatment plan.

Ask a trusted family member or friend to be your advocate.

Know your medications and why you take them. Medication errors are the most common health care errors.

Use a hospital, clinic, surgery center, or other type of health care organization that has undergone a rigorous on-site evaluation against established state-of-the-art quality and safety standards, such as that provided by the Joint Commission.

Participate in all decisions about your treatment. You're the center of the health care team.

Source: Courtesy of The Joint Commission.

New Illnesses and Treatments Emerge. International travel is common, increasing concerns about the spread of diseases. Experts throughout the world respond quickly to emerging illnesses to prevent worldwide spread of disease.

Concern for Prevention of New and Resistant Bacteria Grows. For example, incidences of MRSA (methicillin-resistant *Staphylococcus aureus*) infections increase. Hand sanitizing in all settings is required. Experts voice concern about the overuse of antibiotics.

Bioterrorism and Other Terrorist Attacks Require Being Alert and Prepared. Health care professionals must have plans in place for detecting and responding to bioterrorism, radiation terrorism, and other terrorist attacks early.

Nurses' Roles as Advocates and Leaders Are Key. Nurses play a central role in efficient management of scarce resources (staff, supplies, and equipment). Leadership, critical thinking, delegation, supervision, and organizational and communication skills are essential. New professional practice models emerge to inspire nurses to new heights (Figure 1.3).

Shared Governance and Collaborative Decision Making. We know that shared governance (the inclusion of nurses in making decisions about rules,

NURSING PROFESSIONAL PRACTICE MODEL

P rofessional development

A ccountability

R esearch and quality improvement

T eaching patients and one another

N urses as leaders

R elationships

E xceptional evidence-based practices

S afe patient-centered care focused on outcomes

Making a difference every day

FIGURE 1.3   Professional practice model. The acronym, PARTNERS, gives a good foundation for a professional practice model. Nursing, in partnership with patients and families, clinicians, administrators and educators, collaborate toward the common goal of providing a superior patient experience for patients every day. Each component in the acronym, PARTNERS, is integral to professional nursing practice and shows how nurses collaborate, communicate, and develop professionally. These are also the components needed to give superior patient care. The rising sun represents a new day, every day, while the sun itself symbolizes comfort, energy, light, and something that is ever present. (Adapted with permission from Mainline Hospitals Professional Practice Model © 2010. Available at http://www.mainlinehealth.org/paoli)

procedures, and other aspects of care) gets the best results. (See the Forum for Shared Governance at http://sharedgovernance.org/.)

Shortage of Nurses and Educators Threatens Patient Care. More demands with fewer nurses threaten patient care. Some state laws require more staff for certain types of patients. Nursing and other key players in health care begin to actively recruit people into the profession and make nurses' jobs better. Nurse educators are in demand, as older educators retire with few young educators to replace them.

Preceptors and Mentors Are Valuable Teachers. We recognize the importance of having novices work closely with preceptors and mentors. Preceptors and mentors are experienced nurses with exemplary skills who take the role of teaching and nurturing novices in the clinical setting.

Increasingly Diverse U.S. Population, Nurses, and Students. Many patients, nurses, and students who learned English as a Second Language (ESL) struggle to understand American ways of interacting and learning. Schools and hospitals develop programs to help diverse students and nurses.

Lifelong Learning Required. Speed of change requires commitment to lifelong learning and professional development. Nurses must be knowledgeable workers who are able to make complicated clinical judgments. Independent learning, often through the use of computers and the Internet, is the norm.

Healthy People 2020. Health promotion and disease prevention initiatives aim to improve the nation's health (Box 1.4).

Evidence-Based Care and Best Practices Stressed. Now that we have more research data and know the importance of expert opinion, we continually work to develop the best ways (best practices) to manage specific conditions from outcome and cost perspectives. Today's consumer wants to know the answer to "What evidence do you have that this is the best approach for me?" For information on EBP centers, go to the Agency for Healthcare Research and Quality (AHRQ) Web site at http://www.ahrq.gov/clinic/epc/. The AHRQ is the nation's lead Federal agency for research on health care quality, costs, outcomes, and patient safety.

Case Management, Disease Management, and Telehealth Care Expand. With more people at home and in remote areas with chronic illnesses and complicated treatment regimens, nurses and physicians manage care from a distance, through the use of telephones, television monitors, and other communications technologies. More nurses are involved in disease management, disability management, and case management (care delivery models that aim to keep costs down by helping people with chronic illnesses improve their health status through close monitoring, early intervention, and use of resources).

Box 1.4	Healthy People 2020

Mission
- Identify nationwide health improvement priorities.
- Increase public awareness and understanding of the determinants of health, disease, and disability and the opportunities for progress.
- Provide measurable objectives and goals that are applicable at the national, state, and local levels.
- Engage multiple sectors to take actions to strengthen policies and improve practices that are driven by the best available evidence and knowledge.
- Identify critical research, evaluation, and data collection needs.

Goals
- Attain high-quality, longer lives free of preventable disease, disability, injury, and premature death.
- Achieve health equity, eliminate disparities, and improve the health of all groups.
- Create social and physical environments that promote good health for all.
- Promote quality of life, healthy development, and healthy behaviors across all life stages.

Indicators of Progress
- General Health Status
- Health-Related Quality of Life and Well-Being
- Determinants of Health
- Disparities

Examples of Health Indicators
- Adolescent Health
- Blood Disorders and Blood Safety
- Dementias and Alzheimer's Disease
- Childhood Health
- Genomics
- Global Health
- Health Care-Related Infections
- Health-Related Quality of Life and Well-Being
- Lesbian, Gay, Bisexual, and Transgender Health
- Older Adult Health
- Preparedness
- Sleep Health
- Social Determinants of Health

Source: Summarized from *Healthy People 2020 Framework*. Retrieved November 4, 2011, from http://www. healthypeople.gov/2020/consortium/HP2020Framework.pdf and *What's New for 2020*. Retrieved November 1, 2011, from *http://healthypeople.gov/2020/about/new2020.aspx*.

H.M.O. (HELP ME OUT) ®

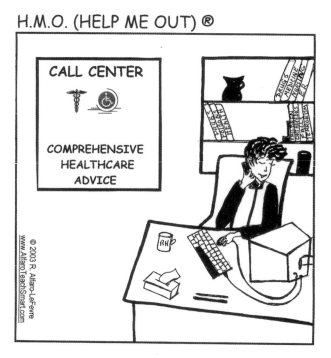

"Take two aspirin, drink lots of fluids, apply heat, get
lots of rest, and bury a potato in the back yard."

Protocols and Critical Paths Guide Care. As we continue to track treatment and outcome data, we have more evidence-based protocols. For example, if you have pneumonia, you'll probably receive a specific antibiotic that's been proven to give the best results and most cost-effective approach. Critical paths (also known as critical pathways, clinical pathways, and care maps), which are standard multidisciplinary plans used to predict and determine care for specific problems, are refined and improved (see example critical path, Appendix A).

More Elderly and Chronically Ill. People live longer with diseases and disabilities. Nurses must focus on promoting health in spite of existing health problems, for example, how to help people with lung disease maximize exercise tolerance. They also must be equipped to deal with patients with multiple health problems, for example, a patient who has diabetes, hypertension, chronic lung disease, and arthritis.

Electronic Health Records (EHR) and Health Information Technology (HIT) Change Health Care Delivery. New technology facilitates diagnosis, decision making, and research. Although these technologies create constant learning challenges, the ultimate improvements save time and improve care quality. Most documentation is done electronically. Smart phones, iPads, and wireless handheld devices enable doctors and nurses to be close at hand, even when far away. On-Line Patient Records (OLPR) promotes accuracy and efficiency.

New Ethical Concerns. Advances in infertility treatment and disease management challenge traditional values regarding conception, birth, death, and dying. Society is very concerned with the ethics of palliative care (care that alleviates pain and suffering and promotes a sense of physical and spiritual well-being, but doesn't cure). Nurses must know how to apply principles of ethics to help patients and families make informed decisions.

Wellness Centers, Holistic and Alternative Therapies. There's a greater focus on promoting health and triggering the body's natural healing powers through holistic and alternative therapies (e.g., diet, exercise, acupuncture, massage, and other ways to manage stress, such as meditation and aromatherapy).

Nurse Wellness Stressed. Many workplaces recognize the need to help nurses stay healthy, giving nurses stress-reduction classes and free (or reduced-cost) wellness center memberships. A healthy nurse is central to safe, efficient nursing care. Concerns about long shifts, patient overloads, and stressful work environments get more attention. New approaches, regulations, and laws continue to address problems like poor nurse–patient ratios and mandatory overtime.

Educated Consumers. Nurses help consumers at both ends of the "knowledge spectrum," from those who are illiterate to those who surf the Internet, becoming experts on the latest information about their problems. Many consumers today are well-informed—often knowing more about their problems than many of those who look after them.

NOTE: The purpose of the critical thinking and clinical reasoning throughout this book is to help you to remember content and practice critical thinking and clinical reasoning skills, not to make you do time-consuming writing exercises. If you don't want to *write* the answers, consider mapping them or discussing them with someone. If you don't need practice, skip the session entirely. The answers in the back of the book are *example responses*—they aren't the *only* answers. They are provided to help you to evaluate and correct your own thinking. If you aren't sure whether your response is acceptable, discuss it with a peer or ask your instructor.

CRITICAL THINKING AND CLINICAL REASONING EXERCISES

1.1 Nursing Process: The Foundation for Clinical Reasoning

Example responses are provided at the end of the book (page 203).

1. Fill in the following blanks: The terms *critical thinking* and *clinical reasoning* are often used (a) _____. *Clinical reasoning* is a specific term that refers to applying the nursing process to assess and (b) _____ patient problems at the point of

care. For reasoning about other clinical issues, such as promoting teamwork and streamlining work flow, nurses usually use (c) _____ _____. Critical thinking is a (d) _____ term that includes clinical reasoning.

2. Using terms a layperson can understand, explain:
   a. The five nursing process phases
   b. Five characteristics of the nursing process that promote safe, effective reasoning.
   c. How the nursing process provides for care that complements care delivered by physicians.

3. Give three reasons why the nursing process is the first tool you need to learn to "think like a nurse."

4. Explain why the accuracy of each step of the nursing process depends on the accuracy of the preceding step.

5. What's wrong with this statement? *He's very good at making diagnoses, but he needs to improve on his assessments.*

6. Suppose you're starting your day looking after a patient who had an appendectomy yesterday. Applying principles of nursing process, what is the *first* thing you should do?

7. Imagine you work in a hospital. Consider the following patient satisfaction issues. Think of three ways you could help nurses stay focused on the things that mean a lot to patients.

Patient Satisfaction: Top 10 Issues

1. Staff sensitivity to the inconvenience that health problems and hospitalizations cause

2. Overall cheerfulness of the hospital

3. Staff concern for patients' privacy

4. Amount of attention paid to patients' special or personal needs

5. Degree to which nurses took patients' health problems seriously

6. Technical skill of nurses

7. Nurses' attitudes toward patients calling them

8. Degree to which the nurses kept patients adequately informed about tests, treatment, and equipment

9. Friendliness of nurses—whether staff is polite to one another

10. Promptness in responding to the call button

Try This on Your Own

With a peer, in a group, or in a personal journal:

1. Discuss the implications of the following statement: Determining your scope of practice means making decisions about what you're legally authorized to assess or do.
2. Address how the code of conduct in Box 1.5 promotes safety, teamwork, and ethical, trusting relationships with patients, families, and other health team members.
3. Get in touch with your feelings about making mistakes. Identify ways you, your patients, and your peers can promote a culture of safety, rather than of blame.
4. Draw a map of how the following concepts are related: critical thinking, clinical reasoning, important thinking needed for any situation, nursing process, thinking at the point of care, patient safety and welfare.
5. Discuss the following online resources:
   - Brent, N. *Protect yourself: Know your nurse practice act.* Available at http://ce.nurse.com/CE548/Protect-Yourself–Know-Your-Nurse-Practice-Act/
   - Gordon, S. (2006). What do nurses really do? *Topics in Advanced Nursing eJournal, 6*(1). Available at http://www.medscape.com/viewarticle/520714_2
   - Frequently asked questions on HIPAA Privacy Rules listed at http://www.hhs.gov/hipaafaq/vs

Box 1.5   Health Team Code of Conduct

As a member of this group/team, I agree to make the following a part of my daily routine.

1. **To keep patient and caregiver safety and welfare as the primary concern in all interactions, including:**
   - Being vigilant and monitoring for care practices that increase risks of errors
   - Remembering no one is perfect and all humans are vulnerable to making mistakes
   - Taking responsibility for being "a safety net" when helping coworkers, anticipating what they may need, and pitching in to prevent mistakes (e.g., "I think that glove is contaminated, let me get you a new one." or "Here's a new needle.")
   - Making it a team principle that "if we witnesses unethical or unsafe practices, it's our responsibility to address it (first directly with the person, then through policies and procedures if warranted)"

2. **To promote empowered partnerships by:**
   - Valuing your time and the contribution you make to the team/group
   - Accepting the diversity in our styles—recognizing that you know yourself best and should be allowed to choose your own approaches

(Continued)

Box 1.5 | **Health Team Code of Conduct (Continued)**

- Promising to be honest, and treating you with respect and courtesy
- Promoting independence and mutual growth by applying the "Platinum Rule" (Treat others as *they* want to be treated, not assuming they have the same desires *you* do)
- Listening openly to new ideas and other perspectives
- Attempting to walk a mile in your shoes
- Committing to resolving conflict without resorting to using power
- Taking responsibility for my own emotional well-being (if I feel bad about something, it's my responsibility to do something about it)
- Ensuring that we both:
  - Stay focused on our joint purpose and responsibilities for achieving it
  - Make decisions together as much as possible
  - Realize that we're accountable for the outcomes (consequences) of our actions
  - Have the right to say no, so long as it doesn't mean neglecting responsibilities

3. **To foster open communication and a positive work environment by:**
   - Addressing specific issues and behaviors
   - Acknowledging/apologizing if I've caused inconvenience or made a mistake
   - Doing my "homework" before drawing conclusions
   - Maintaining confidentiality when I'm used as a sounding board
   - Using only ONE person as my sounding board before I decide to either give feedback or drop the issue
   - Validating any rumors I hear
   - Redirecting coworkers who are talking about someone to speak directly to the person
   - Addressing unsafe or unethical behavior directly and according to policies
   - Offering feedback as indicated:
     - Within 72 hours, using "I" statements ("I feel..." rather than "You make me feel...")
     - Describing behaviors and giving specific examples
     - Limiting discussion to the event at hand and not discussing past history and telling you honestly and openly the impact of the behavior

4. **To be approachable and open to feedback by:**
   - Taking responsibility for my actions and words
   - Taking time to reflect on what was said, rather than blaming, defending, or rejecting
   - Asking for clarification of the perceived behaviors
   - Remembering that there's always a little bit of truth in every criticism
   - Staying focused on what I can learn from the situation

Source: © 2012 R. Alfaro-LeFevre. Available at www.AlfaroTeachSmart.com.

DEVELOPING CRITICAL THINKING AND CLINICAL REASONING SKILLS

Developing reasoning skills is like developing other complex skills: as you practice and gain experience, these skills become automatic—you develop thinking habits that will serve you and your patients well. The exercises throughout this book are designed to help you develop, refine, and practice critical thinking and clinical reasoning abilities. As you complete each chapter, learning to apply the principles and rules of the nursing process, you'll begin to develop habits that help you be more automatic when reasoning in nursing situations.

Critical Thinking Indicators

Boxes 1.6, 1.7, and 1.8 list Critical Thinking Indicators (CTIs). CTIs are behaviors that evidence suggests promote critical thinking in nursing. Remember that *critical thinking* is a broad term that includes *clinical reasoning*. Keep in mind that no one is perfect and abilities vary with experience and familiarity with the people and circumstances involved. Also realize that CTIs may change, depending on specialty practice.

RULE   **Critical thinking and clinical reasoning are contextual—they change with circumstances (one size doesn't fit all).** Look for changes *in the patient or situation* that require you to change your approach. For example, if you go from working in a hospital (where you're in charge and equipment and resources are plentiful) to working in home care (where you're a guest in someone else's home and have to improvise), you may have to rethink the whole process.

Get a beginning idea of where you stand in relation to being a critical thinker—consider each indicator in boxes and rate your abilities, using the following 0–10 scale.

0 = I'm not very good at demonstrating this indicator.
10 = I almost always demonstrate this indicator.

While CTIs are listed separately, they're interrelated. For example, simply having knowledge (Box 1.7) doesn't indicate critical thinking. It's the ability to *apply* knowledge to accomplish intellectual skills (Box 1.8) that indicates critical thinking.

The 4-Circle CT Model

Another way to look at critical thinking is to use the four circles shown in Figure 1.4 to get a "picture" of what it takes to think critically.

Going clockwise on the circles, here's what you need to do:

1. **Develop CT attitudes, characteristics, and behaviors** (top circle). When you develop personal CT characteristics like the ones Box 1.6, the skills in the other circles come readily.

(text continues after Figure 1.4, page 33)

Box 1.6 Personal Critical Thinking Indicators (CTIs)

Note: **Personal CTIs are brief descriptions of behaviors that demonstrate characteristics that promote critical thinking. The below is the ideal. No one is perfect.**

- **Self-aware:** Identifies own learning, personality, and communication style preferences; clarifies biases, strengths, and limitations; acknowledges when thinking may be influenced by emotions or self-interest.
- **Genuine/authentic:** Shows true self; demonstrates behaviors that indicate stated values.
- **Effective communicator:** Listens well (shows deep understanding of others' thoughts, feelings, and circumstances); speaks and writes with clarity (gets key points across to others).
- **Curious and inquisitive:** Asks questions; looks for reasons, explanations, and meaning; seeks new information to broaden understanding.
- **Alert to context:** Looks for changes in circumstances that warrant a need to modify approaches; investigates thoroughly when situations warrant precise, in-depth thinking.
- **Analytical and insightful:** Identifies relationships; expresses deep understanding.
- **Logical and intuitive:** Draws reasonable conclusions (if this is so, then it follows that …because…); uses intuition as a guide; acts on intuition only with knowledge of risks involved.
- **Confident and resilient:** Expresses faith in ability to reason and learn; overcomes problems and disappointments.
- **Honest and upright:** Looks for the truth, even if it sheds unwanted light; demonstrates integrity (adheres to moral and ethical standards; admits flaws in thinking).
- **Autonomous/responsible:** Self-directed, self-disciplined, and accepts accountability.
- **Careful and prudent:** Seeks help as needed; suspends or revises judgment as indicated by new or incomplete data
- **Open and fair-minded:** Shows tolerance for different viewpoints; questions how own viewpoints are influencing thinking.
- **Sensitive to diversity:** Expresses appreciation of human differences related to values, culture, personality, or learning style preferences; adapts to preferences when feasible.
- **Creative:** Offers alternative solutions and approaches; comes up with useful ideas.
- **Realistic and practical:** Admits when things aren't feasible; looks for useful solutions.
- **Reflective and self-corrective:** Carefully considers meaning of data and interpersonal interactions, asks for feedback; corrects own thinking, alert to potential errors by self and others, finds ways to avoid future mistakes.
- **Proactive:** Anticipates consequences, plans ahead, acts on opportunities.
- **Courageous:** Stands up for beliefs, advocates for others, doesn't hide from challenges.
- **Patient and persistent:** Waits for right moment; perseveres to achieve best results.
- **Flexible:** Changes approaches as needed to get the best results.
- **Health-oriented:** Promotes a healthy lifestyle; uses healthy behaviors to manage stress.
- **Improvement-oriented (self, patients, systems):** **Self**—Identifies learning needs; finds ways to overcome limitations, seeks out new knowledge. **Patients**—Promotes health; maximizes function, comfort, and convenience. **Systems**—Identifies risks and problems with health care systems; promotes safety, quality, satisfaction, and cost containment.

Source: Alfaro-LeFevre, R. (2012). *Critical thinking indicators.* Available at www.AlfaroTeachSmart.com. All rights reserved. No use without permission.

Box 1.7	**Knowledge Critical Thinking Indicators (CTIs) (Requirements Vary, Depending on Specialty Practice)**

Clarifies Nursing Knowledge
- Nursing and medical terminology
- Nursing versus medical and other models, roles, and responsibilities
- Scope of nursing practice (qualifications; applicable standards, laws, and rules and regulations)
- Related anatomy, physiology, and pathophysiology
- Spiritual, social, and cultural concepts
- Normal and abnormal growth and development (pediatric, adult, and gerontologic implications)
- Normal and abnormal function (bio-psycho-social-cultural-spiritual)
- Factors affecting normal function (bio-psycho-social-cultural-spiritual)
- Nutrition and pharmacology principles
- Behavioral health and disease management
- Signs and symptoms of common problems and complications
- Nursing process, nursing theories, research, and evidence-based practice
- Reasons behind policies, procedures and interventions; diagnostic studies implications
- Ethical and legal principles
- Risk management and infection control
- Safety standards, healthy workplace standards, and principles of learning and safety cultures
- Interrelationship of health care disciplines and systems
- Reliable information resources

Demonstrates
- Focused nursing assessment skills (e.g., breath sounds or IV site assessment)
- Mathematical problem solving for drug calculations
- Related technical skills (e.g., n/g tube or other equipment management)

Clarifies Knowledge of Self
- Personal biases, values, beliefs, needs
- How own culture, thinking, personality, and learning style preferences differ from others'
- Level of commitment to organizational mission and values

Source: Alfaro-LeFevre, R. (2012). *Critical thinking indicators.* Available at www.AlfaroTeachSmart.com. All rights reserved. No use without permission.

Box 1.8

Intellectual Skills Critical Thinking Indicators (Behaviors Demonstrating Intellectual Competencies)

Nursing Process and Decision-Making Skills

- Communicates effectively orally and in writing
- Identifies practice scope; applies standards, principles, laws, and ethics codes
- Makes safety and infection control a priority; prevents and deals with mistakes constructively
- Includes patient, family, and key stakeholders in decision making; teaches patient, self, and others
- Identifies purpose and focus of assessment
- Assesses systematically and comprehensively.
- Distinguishes normal from abnormal; identifies risks for abnormal
- Distinguishes relevant from irrelevant; clusters relevant data together
- Identifies assumptions and inconsistencies; checks accuracy and reliability (validates data)
- Recognizes missing information; gains more data as needed.
- Concludes what's known and unknown; draws reasonable conclusions—gives evidence to support them
- Identifies both problems and their underlying cause(s) and related factors; includes patient and family perspectives
- Recognizes changes in patient status; takes appropriate action
- Considers multiple ideas, explanations, and solutions
- Determines individualized outcomes and uses them to plan and give care
- Manages risks, predicts complications
- Weighs risks and benefits; anticipates consequences and implications—individualizes interventions accordingly
- Sets priorities and makes decisions in a timely way
- Reassesses to monitor outcomes (responses)
- Promotes health, function, comfort, and well-being
- Identifies ethical issues and takes appropriate action
- Uses human and information resources; detects bias

Additional Skills

- Advocates for patients, self, and others
- Establishes empowered partnerships with patients, families, peers, and coworkers
- Fosters positive interpersonal relationships; addresses conflicts fairly; promotes healthy workplace and learning cultures
- Promotes teamwork (focuses on common goals, respects diversity; encourages others to contribute in their own way)
- Facilitates and navigates change
- Organizes and manages time and environment
- Gives and takes constructive criticism
- Delegates appropriately (matches patient needs with worker competencies; determines worker learning needs, supervises and teaches as indicated; monitors results personally)
- Leads, inspires, and helps others move toward common goals
- Demonstrates systems thinking (shows awareness of relationships existing within and across health care systems)

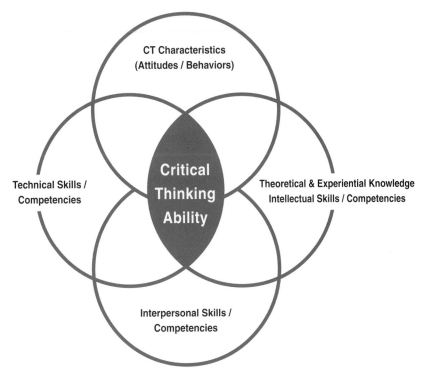

FIGURE 1.4 The 4-circle critical thinking (CT) model. (© 2012 R. Alfaro-LeFevre. www.Alfaro TeachSmart.com)

2. **Acquire theoretical and experiential knowledge and intellectual skills.**
3. **Gain interpersonal skills.** If you can't get along with others, you will be unlikely to think critically because you will soon be out of the loop (people will avoid you). At the other end of the spectrum, if you're "too nice" to confront or give criticism, you contribute little to others' critical thinking and often lose brainpower to stress. Developing interpersonal skills is as important as developing clinical skills. Table 1.3 (next page) lists behaviors affecting interpersonal relationships.
4. **Practice technical skills.** Until technical skills (e.g., IV skills or computer skills) are second nature, you have less brain power for critical thinking (due to the "brain drain" of mastering technical skills).

Using Simulation and Debriefing

As you can see from the 4-Circle CT Model, developing clinical reasoning is complex, takes time, and best comes with hands-on experience on the job over time. But, because we must keep patient safety top priority, using simulated experiences before hands-on learning in the clinical setting is a great way to develop clinical reasoning skills. Simulated experience—a powerful way to learn because you can make (and recover from) mistakes in a safe environment—continues to evolve with technology that makes the experience as close to reality as possible. Honest dialogue in

Table 1.3 Behaviors Affecting Interpersonal Relationships

Behaviors That Enhance Interpersonal Relationships	Behaviors That Inhibit Interpersonal Relationships
Conveying an attitude of openness, acceptance, and lack of prejudice.	Conveying an attitude of doubt, mistrust, or negative judgment.
Being honest.	Being deceptive.
Taking initiative and responsibility; responding to others' concerns.	Conveying an "it's not my job" attitude.
Being reliable.	Not meeting commitments, only partially meeting commitments, or not being punctual.
Demonstrating humility.	Demonstrating self-importance.
Showing respect for what others are, have been, or may become.	"Talking down" or assuming familiarity.
Accepting accountability.	Making excuses or placing blame where it doesn't belong.
Showing genuine interest.	Acting like you're only doing something because it's a job.
Conveying appreciation for others' time.	Assuming others have more time than we do.
Accepting expression of positive *and* negative feelings.	Showing anger when negative feelings are expressed.
Being frank and forthright.	Sending mixed messages, saying things just because we think it's what the other person seems to want to hear, or talking behind others' backs.
Admitting when we've been wrong.	Denying or ignoring when we've made an error.
Apologizing if we've caused distress or inconvenience.	Acting like nothing happened or making excuses.
Being willing to forgive and forget.	Holding grudges.
Showing a positive attitude.	Conveying an "it'll never work" attitude.
Conveying a sense of humor.	Acting like there's no room for anything but "serious business."
Allowing others control.	Trying to control others.
Giving credit where credit is due.	Ignoring achievements or taking credit that doesn't belong to us.

debriefing sessions after simulation is an important part of simulation because you can talk objectively about what went well, what issues you had, how you could be more prepared, and what to do if those issues arise in real situations.

WILLINGNESS AND ABILITY TO CARE

Develop critical thinking skills means making a commitment to be willing and able to care. Caring is so central to nursing that's that it's integrated throughout the NCLEX test plan.[2] Consider Box 1.9, which shows how caring is described on NCLEX and by Jean Watson, a pioneer in the science of caring.

Willingness to Care

Being willing to care means making the choice to do what it takes to help others. This includes choosing to

- Keep the focus on what's best for the consumer (patient, family, community)
- Respect the values, beliefs, and individuality of others
- Stay involved, even when problems become chronic or more complex
- Maintain a healthy lifestyle so you're able to help

Box 1.9 | **Caring as Addressed by NCLEX® and Watson**

NCLEX
Caring **is interaction of the nurse and client in an atmosphere of mutual respect and trust**. In this collaborative environment, the nurse provides encouragement, hope, support, and compassion to help achieve desired outcomes.

Jean Watson
- The practice of caring is central to nursing.
- Caring responses accept a person not only as he or she is now but as what he or she may become.
- Effective caring promotes health and individual or family growth.
- Caring is more "healthogenic" than is curing—science of caring is complementary to the science of curing.
- Caring can be effectively demonstrated and practiced only interpersonally.
- Caring consists of carative factors that result in the satisfaction of certain human needs.
- A caring environment promotes development of potential while allowing people to choose the best action for themselves at a given point in time.

Source: National Council of State Boards of Nursing 2010 NCLEX-RN Test Plan. Retrieved July 1, 2011, from https://www.ncsbn.org/1287.htm
Source: Watson, J. (2001). Jean Watson: Theory of human caring. In M. E. Parker (Ed.), *Nursing theories and nursing practice* (pp. 343–354). Philadelphia: F. A. Davis Company.
Source: Watson, J. (2002). Instruments for assessing and measuring caring in nursing and health sciences. New York: Springer.

Being willing to care also means making a commitment to make the following professional behaviors part of your everyday practice.

ANA Professional Practice Behaviors

As a nurse, you're accountable for the following professional behaviors.[1]

- Maintain knowledge, skills, and competence in current practices
- Evaluate the quality and effectiveness of your own performance and of nursing practice in relation to professional standards and rules and regulations
- Practice collegially, contributing to the professional development of peers and colleagues
- Collaborate with patients, families, peers, professionals, and others
- Integrate research findings into practice
- Use resources to improve safety, effectiveness, cost, and impact on planning and giving care.

Being Able to Care

Being able to care requires taking care of ourselves, understanding ourselves (being self-aware), and understanding others.

Understanding Ourselves

Because our tendencies, reactions, and habits tend to change as we grow and mature, gaining deep understanding of ourselves is a lifelong pursuit. When we learn about ourselves and recognize how our values and frame of reference influence our thinking and ability to understand others, we can take deliberate steps to be more objective and helpful.

Understanding Others

Understanding others takes active empathetic listening—being fully present and working to fully comprehend someone else's perceptions. It's like trying to "view the world through someone else's glasses" or "walk a mile in another's shoes." It requires active, focused listening as described in the following section.

Listening Actively and Empathetically

Consider the following steps, and then decide how you can apply them to the case scenario in Box 1.10 (next page).

1. Eliminate thoughts about how you, yourself, see the situation.
2. Listen carefully for *feelings*, trying to identify with how the other person perceives his situation. Don't allow yourself to think about how *you* feel or how you're going to respond; think only about the content of what you're hearing.
3. Reflect on what you heard; then name the feelings that were expressed.

Box 1.10 | **Case Scenario: Empathetic Listening Promotes Therapeutic Communication and Understanding**

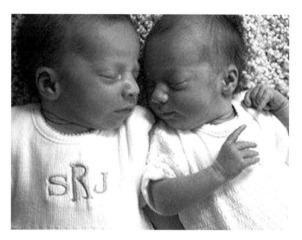

© 2007 J. Riley.

Today Pat is caring for Sharon, who just gave birth to healthy twin girls. Pat herself has always wanted children but has been unable to conceive. Pat notes that Sharon seems very quiet. Recognizing the importance of being an active, empathetic listener, Pat has the following conversation with Sharon.

- **Pat:** "You've been pretty quiet since I came on."
- **Sharon:** "I can't help it. I'm supposed to be happy, but I'm sad. I wanted to have at least one boy."
- **Pat (makes a conscious effort to eliminate personal thoughts about the fact that this woman is crying over twin girls, when she, herself, has never been able to have *one* child—then rephrases what she heard):** "You're supposed to be happy, but you feel sad?"
- **Sharon:** "Yes."
- **Pat:** (Uses silence to reflect on the feeling of sadness and encourage Sharon to continue)
- **Sharon:** "The doctor told us one of the babies was a boy. I planned to name him after my father. My Dad is dying and I wanted to do this for him."
- **Pat (connects to what Sharon must be feeling):** "That *would* be a disappointment."
- **Sharon (crying):** "Yes. I had it all pictured in my mind."
- **Pat:** (Stays quiet, conveys acceptance and understanding as Sharon cries.)
- **Pat (detaches and becomes logical and objective):** "Sharon, I know you feel sad right now. Hormones may be influencing how you feel. But, you have two beautiful little girls waiting to see you. Maybe we can figure out a girl's name that's a version of your father's. Shall I go get them?"
- **Sharon (smiling):** "Yes. I only held them for a few minutes. I have to admit that it will be fun dressing two girls."

4. Seek verification that you understood the message and the feelings correctly. Keep trying until you're sure you understand.

5. Detach, come back to your own frame of reference. Try to separate yourself from the emotions involved so that you can stay logical and objective.

CRITICAL THINKING AND CLINICAL REASONING EXERCISES

1.2   **Developing Critical Thinking and Clinical Reasoning Skills**

Example responses are provided at the end of the book (pages 203–204).

1. Fill in the following blanks:

   Developing critical thinking and clinical reasoning skills is like developing other (a) _____ skills: if you practice, they become habits of your (b) _____.

2. How are the critical thinking indicators in Boxes 1.6, 1.7, and 1.8 related to the circles in the 4-Circle CT Model (Figure 1.4)?

3. What is the relationship between the knowledge CTIs (Box 1.7) and the intellectual skills CTIs (Box 1.8)?

Try This on Your Own

In a personal journal, with a peer, or in a group:

1. Discuss how the following statements from *Nursing's Social Policy Statement*[9] relate to this chapter.
   - Health and illness are human experiences.
   - The presence of illness does not preclude health, nor does optimal health preclude illness.
   - An essential feature of contemporary nursing practice is the provision of a caring relationship that facilitates healing.
   - Humans manifest an essential unity of mind, body, and spirit.
   - Human experience is contextually and culturally defined.

2. Imagine you'll be looking after a 71-year-old man the day after gallbladder surgery. He has a nasogastric tube and an IV attached to a pump. He also has a history of congestive heart failure (CHF). Draw the 4-Circle Model, then apply it to decide the skills you need to have to care for this man.

3. Discuss your personal experiences with the following caring behaviors.

Caring Behaviors

- Acknowledge that each person's experience is unique (don't assume you know—or make negative judgments about—others' feelings).

- Monitor patients closely and let them know you're doing it (e.g., "I'll check on you every 15 minutes").
- Keep people informed—listen actively and speak compassionately.
- Instill hope (creating a vision of what "can be").
- Offer companionship—just sit quietly.
- Avoid clichés (e.g., "God gives you only what you can bear").
- Help people to stay in touch with positive aspects of their lives (e.g., ask about friends, pets, special interests, or hobbies).
- Give patients and families resources to help themselves.

4. Improve your interpersonal skills. Learn about your innate personality and how to get along with "difficult" people. Read *Don't Worry! Be Happy! Harmonize Diversity Through Personality Sensitivity*, available at http://ce.nurse.com/ce236-60/dont-worry-be-happy-harmonize-diversity-through-personality-sensitivity/

5. Practice empathetic listening. Ask someone to tell you about an upsetting experience in his or her childhood. Use the steps of listening empathetically as discussed in this chapter.

6. In a personal journal, with a peer, or in a group, discuss the implications of the following Voices and Think About It entries.

Voices

Why We Have Two Hands
"God gave us two hands: One to help others and the other to help ourselves."[10]
—Eileen Lupton, RN, BSN

Where Nurses Stand
"Nurses stand at the intersection of all activity."[11]
—Tim Porter-O'Grady, DM, EdD, ScD(h), FAAN

Who Guards the Patient?
"Safety lies at the crux of the care we deliver. And yet we all know that there are so many factors that affect patient safety—from communication snafus through systems design problems through inadequate staffing... Nurses are in pivotal roles within health care settings because they coordinate, implement, and evaluate the patient care that is administered by the entire team on an ongoing basis."[12]
—Rebecca B. Rice, RN, EdD, MPH

Six Golden Rules for Nurses
1. Everybody knows something.
2. No one knows everything.
3. In light of rules #1 and #2, create a colleague-supportive environment. Share what you know. Teach one another. Answer questions. Ask questions. There's no such thing as a stupid question, but we've all asked it!

4. One nurse shouldn't have a horrible day unless all nurses are having a horrible day.
5. One nurse shouldn't have a breeze of a day unless all nurses are having a breeze of a day.
6. **Work as a team.** Help one another with the physical demands of the work. You're responsible for your own patients, but you're responsible to each other as nurses and human beings. When you help one another, the *patients* benefit!

Source: Adapted from Agostino, P. (2000). *Ten Golden Rules for Nurses.* Retrieved November 1, 2011, from http://news.nurse.com/apps/pbcs.dll/article?AID=20001100306

 ## Think About It

Patient-Centered Care—"Nothing About Me Without Me"

The phrase "nothing about me without me" was first used by an English midwife and has since been used by many authors. Patients and family caregivers must key players in decision making. When you provide information and encourage people to take an active role in their plan of care, you empower them to maximize health and open the door to patient satisfaction and health care efficiency.

Learn how to establish partnerships with mutual trust. Move from an *I'll-take-care-of-you* approach to one that sends the message, *I want you to know what to do when I'm not here.* Assume that patients know themselves well. Involve them by using comments like "You know yourself best—tell me what you'd like to see happen," "What's most important to you?" and "I want you to be able to make informed choices—we share a common purpose and we're both responsible for what happens."

Nurses Are Stewards for Safe Passage

Just as a ship's steward protects passengers on a journey, your job as a nurse is to protect patients and help them navigate safe passage through the health care system. You hold patients' lives in your hands, but they are the ones who should be "at the helm, directing where they want to go." Involve patients and families early in decision making. Ask questions like, "What are the main things you want to accomplish?" Help patients understand the concept of stewardship by saying something like "I'm here to take care of you, but more importantly, I'm here to make sure you know how to take care of yourself when I'm not here"... "Let me know when you have questions or concerns"... "Stay involved in your care—you know yourself best and will do better if you let us know what you need and want."

Cutting Costs, Not Corners

Cutting costs doesn't mean "cutting corners." It means working to get *equal results within a budget.* For example, ask the pharmacist whether a generic antibiotic that is taken five times a day can be substituted for a more costly brand-name drug that is taken only three times a day. On the other hand, if you don't get the results you want because it's too inconvenient to take the generic drug five times a day, point out that it may be cheaper in the long run to use the more expensive brand drug. (Physician approval is required.)

Are You Culturally Competent?

Being culturally competent does not mean that you must know the beliefs of *every* culture—no one can know it all. It means that you need to learn about the values, beliefs, and customs of the populations you work with *most*. Get help when you find yourself caring for patients and families who are of a culture that you know little about. Even when you're familiar with a certain groups' beliefs, you must avoid making assumptions. For example, most Amish people don't use electricity or technology. Yet, today, some Amish people have cell phones and leaf blowers. Work to develop your cultural competence: (1) Get in touch with your own values and beliefs. Understand how these affect your ability to give nursing care. (2) Work to understand, value, and incorporate your patients' cultural needs into the plan of care. (3) Don't make assumptions, as each person is unique within a cultural group. Ask patients to tell you if they have any particular beliefs or traditions that you should incorporate into the plan of care.

You Don't Learn to Swim in the Living Room

Knowledge and experience are the two main things you need to develop clinical reasoning skills. The adage "practice makes perfect" rings true for everyone. Seek out real and simulated experiences to help you become the nurse you want to be. Work to make your experiences as real as possible. As Elizabeth Smart—who was kidnapped as a child and now teaches survival skills—says, "You don't learn to swim in the living room."

This Chapter and NCLEX*

1. **The following processes are integrated throughout:**
   - Nursing process (Assessment, Diagnosis, Planning, Implementation, and Evaluation)
   - Caring
   - Teaching and learning
   - Communication and documentation
2. **Tests the following categories:**
   - Safe, effective care environment—management of care (16%–22% of the test)
   - Safe, effective care environment—safety and infection control (8%–14% of the test)
   - Health promotion and maintenance (6%–12% of the test)
   - Psychosocial integrity (6%–12% of the test)
   - Physiologic integrity (around 50% of the test), including basic care and comfort and assistance in performance of ADL (6%–12% of the test), pharmacology and intravenous (IV) therapy (13%–19% of the test), risk reduction (10%–16% of the test), and physiologic adaptation (11%–17% of the test).
3. **Most questions are multiple-choice** requiring you to select one answer; there are a few "alternate item questions" that require you to select one or more responses, fill in the blank (including calculation and prioritizing questions), or click and drag the mouse to select a "hot spot." All items may include charts, tables, or graphs.
4. **The test plan is based on the results of the RN Practice Analysis** that was conducted in 2008, evaluated in 2009, and implemented in April 2010.

*The author acknowledges the help of Judith Miller (http://judymillernclexreview.com) and Deanne Blach (www.DeanneBlach.com) in developing NCLEX content throughout this book. Source: National Council of State Boards of Nursing 2010 NCLEX-RN Test Plan. Retrieved November 1, 2011, from https://www.ncsbn.org/1287.htm

5. **Includes questions on all major specialties,** as well as advance directives, family systems, cultural diversity, error prevention, bioterrorism, disaster response, human sexuality, and mental health. Expect questions on the following:
   - Applying principles of infection control (e.g., hand hygiene, aseptic/sterile technique)
   - Providing care within the legal scope of practice
   - Maintaining patient confidentiality
   - Ensuring proper patient identification
   - Protecting patients from injury (falls, malfunctioning equipment, electrical hazards)
   - Practicing in a manner consistent with a code of ethics
   - Reviewing pertinent data prior to medication administration
   - Preparing and giving medications applying the rights of medication administration
   - Prioritizing workload to manage time effectively
   - Using approved abbreviations and standard terminology when documenting care
   - Managing care of patient receiving peritoneal dialysis
   - Providing intrapartum care and education
   - Facilitating group sessions
   - Identifying and reporting occupational/environmental exposures
   - Providing care and support for patients with non–substance-related dependencies

Key Points

- The nursing process is the foundation for clinical reasoning, required by national practice standards, tested on NCLEX, and the first tool you need to learn to "think like a nurse." It's a *cycle*—rather than a linear process—and is purposeful, humanistic, systematic, organized, dynamic, and outcome-focused (results-oriented).
- The five steps—*Assessment, Diagnosis, Planning, Implementation*, and *Evaluation (ADPIE)*—overlap and are interrelated. The accuracy of all of the steps depends on good communication skills and factual, relevant, and comprehensive assessment data.
- The nursing process is more than something that guides formal care planning and documentation—it's what should guide your thinking at the point of care every day.
- The terms CT and CR are often used interchangeably. CR is a specific term that refers to the assessment and management of patient problems at the point of care (applying

nursing process). For reasoning about other issues such as promoting teamwork and streamlining work flow, nurses usually use the term CT. CT is a *broad term* that includes CR.
- The nursing process complements what other health care professionals do by focusing on both the medical problems and on the *impact* of medical problems and treatment plans on patients' lives (human responses). The nursing process also aims to promote health by maximizing independence, sense of well-being, and ability to function, regardless of the presence of illness or disability.
- Using the nursing process requires you to apply national and state laws and local policies and procedures. It also requires following ethics codes and principles, and applying a code of conduct (Box 1.5).
- Being competent in using the nursing process requires a commitment to develop critical thinking behaviors (Boxes 1.6, 1.7, and 1.8), strong interpersonal and technical skills, and

APPLYING NURSING PROCESS PRINCIPLES
AS DESCRIBED IN THIS BOOK

THINKING CRITICALLY ABOUT PATIENT CARE

☐ Follow standards, policies, procedures, ethics codes, and laws (state practice acts).
☐ Communicate effectively (listen, speak, and chart carefully).
☐ Promote independence, function, comfort and well-being (as defined by patients themselves); guard patient privacy.
☐ Partner with patients, colleagues, and stakeholders to clarify expected outcomes and make decisions.
☐ Assess systematically—draw conclusions based on *facts*.
☐ Address bio-psycho-social-cultural-spiritual needs.
☐ Access information—apply knowledge and evidence.
☐ Remember that laws prohibit you from making medical diagnoses independently; but that *you* are *accountable* for reporting signs and symptoms and activating the chain of command as needed.
☐ Change your approach depending on the patient and situation (critical thinking is contextual and changes with circumstances).
☐ Perform interventions (assess, re-assess, revise, record).
☐ Monitor (evaluate) outcomes.
☐ Keep patients safe (teach patients to speak up; report error-prone systems, follow safety procedures).
☐ Think ahead, think in action, think back (reflect on your thinking).
☐ Be accountable and responsible—improve care practices and your own knowledge and performance.

FIGURE 1.5   Applying nursing process principles to think critically about patient care.

being willing and able to care. The 4-Circle CT model (Fig. 1.3) gives you a picture of what it takes to think critically.

● Figure 1.5 summarizes strategies to use the nursing process as described in this chapter.

● Scan this chapter for important rules and illustrations, then compare where you stand in relation to the Expected Learning Outcomes in the chapter opener (page 2).

References

1. American Nurses Association. (2010). *Nursing scope and standards of performance and standards of clinical practice* (2nd ed.). Silver Springs, MD: nursesbooks.org.
2. National Council of State Boards of Nursing. (2010). NCLEX-RN Test Plan. Retrieved November 3, 2011, from https://www.ncsbn.org/1287.htm
3. Alfaro-LeFevre, R. (2013). *Critical thinking, clinical reasoning, and clinical judgment: A practical approach* (5th ed.). Philadelphia: Saunders-Elsevier.
4. Buppert, C. (2008). The legal distinction between the practice of medicine and the practice of nursing. *The Journal for Nurse Practitioners, 4*(1), 22–24.

5. Institute of Medicine. (2000). *To err is human: Building a safer health system*. Washington, DC: National Academies Press. Retrieved November 5, 2011, from The National Academies Press Web site: www.nap.edu/openbook.php?isbn=0309068371

6. Quality and Safety Education for Nurses (QSEN) goal statement. Retrieved November, 2011, from www.QSEN.org

7. Alfaro-LeFevre, R. (2012). Evidenced-based Critical Thinking Indicators. Retrieved November 5 from www.AlfaroTeachSmart.com

8. American Nurses Association. (2008). *Guide to code of ethics for nurses*. Washington, DC: American Nurses Publishing.

9. American Nurses Association. (2010). *Nursing's social policy statement: The essence of the profession* (3rd ed.). Silver Springs, MD: Author.

10. Lupton, E. (2004). Unpublished essay submitted for application to Villanova University College of Nursing.

11. Porter-O'Grady, T. Email communication. November, 2010.

12. Rice, R. B. (2003). Patient safety: Who guards the patient? *Online Journal of Issues in Nursing, 8*(3), 1. Retrieved June 28, 2011, from www.nursingworld.org

Chapter 2
Assessment

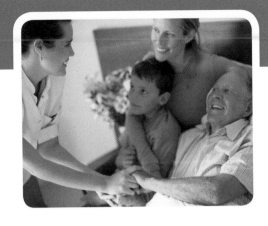

What's in This Chapter?

Stressing that the safety and efficiency of all steps of the nursing process depend on the accuracy and completeness of *Assessment*, this chapter addresses how to do an assessment that's tailored to each specific patient situation (one size doesn't fit all). You learn what an assessment that promotes sound clinical reasoning "looks like" and how to use standard and electronic tools to guide and record your assessments. You learn how to set priorities during assessment, develop the knowledge and skills needed to make clinical decisions, and think your way through NCLEX and other tests. You also get detailed guidelines for interviewing and examining patients and study how to complete six dynamic and interrelated phases of assessment: (1) collecting data; (2) identifying cues and making inferences; (3) validating data; (4) clustering related data; (5) identifying patterns/testing first impressions; and (6) reporting and recording data.

ANA Standards Related to This Chapter

Standard 1   **Assessment.** The registered nurse collects comprehensive data pertinent to the health care consumer's health and/or situation.[1]

Critical Thinking and Clinical Reasoning Exercises

Exercises 2.1   Developing Your Interview and Physical Assessment Skills
Exercises 2.2   Subjective and Objective Data; Cues and Inferences; Validating Data
Exercises 2.3   Clustering Related Data
Exercises 2.4   Reporting and Recording Significant Data

Expected Learning Outcomes

After studying this chapter, you should be able to:

1. Describe six characteristics of an assessment that promotes critical thinking, including why each one promotes critical thinking.

2. Clarify the relationships among the six phases of assessment (collecting data; identifying cues and making inferences; validating (verifying) data; clustering related data; identifying patterns/testing first impressions; reporting and recording data).

3. Discuss what can happen in the other steps of the nursing process if *Assessment* is incomplete or incorrect.

4. Explain why using evidence-based standard tools doesn't replace the need for you to develop independent critical thinking skills.

5. Compare and contrast the terms *data base assessment, focus assessment*, and *quick priority assessment*.

6. Apply ethical, cultural, and spiritual considerations to performing assessments.

7. Describe nurses' responsibilities in relation to assessing for disease, disability, and risk management.

8. Refine your interviewing skills, including knowing when and how to use open-ended questions, closed-ended questions, and exploratory statements.

9. Develop your physical assessments skills, including how to prioritize your assessment and gain information that clarifies information gained from your patient interview.

10. Identify subjective and objective data in a nursing assessment, explaining why both are needed.

11. Identify cues and make inferences (draw conclusions) based on evidence from patient assessment data.

12. Explain why clustering data in more than one way (e.g., both a body systems model and a nursing model) promotes critical thinking.

13. Decide what information to report and record the next time you're in the clinical setting.

14. Explain how to use the *Read Back Rule*, the *Repeat Back Rule*, and *SBAR* approach for communicating patient care.

ASSESSMENT: THE KEY TO SAFETY, ACCURACY, AND EFFICIENCY

Assessment—the first step to determining health status and identifying actual and potential problems—is the foundation for all the other phases of nursing process. It's the key to safety, accuracy, and efficiency. Whenever you're in a new setting—for instance, if you move from a medical-surgical unit to a behavioral health unit—the first thing you need to do is to develop sound assessment skills. Whenever a question on NCLEX or other tests asks you *What should you do first?*, the correct response is often something related to assessment.

RULE   **At every phase of the nursing process, remember: Assess the patient first.** Patient status changes. Your direct assessment is the "last line of defense" to ensure that information is correct and planned care is safe and appropriate.

While electronic records and health information technology play an important part in assessment by jogging your mind what to assess, this chapter teaches you principles you need to have *in your head* to collect, prioritize, and *think* about the data you gather. It helps you develop habits that promote an organized, factual, and complete assessment.

As you read through this chapter, keep in mind that the main purpose of assessment is to gain all the information needed to:

1. Identify, prevent, and treat health problems
2. Promote optimum functioning, independence, and well-being
3. Determine individualized patient outcomes

Also remember from Chapter 1 that what you're legally authorized to assess is determined by your scope of practice.

Let's start by reviewing the diagram from Chapter 1 that shows *Assessment* and *Diagnosis* as overlapping phases.

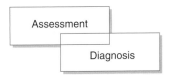

It's not unusual to find that as you *assess* (first box in the preceding diagram) you begin to get *an idea* of the *diagnoses* (second box). This should prompt you to focus your assessment to gain more information to decide if the diagnoses and problems you suspect are indeed present. For example, if the data make you suspect an infection, you work to gain more information to decide whether or not signs and symptoms of infection are present. Sometimes, you may even "work backwards": you know your patient's problems and you assess the patient to determine the status of the problems. You may also be asked to screen patients for a specific problem (e.g., *depression*), and you do an assessment to decide whether or not the problem is present.

ASSESSMENTS THAT PROMOTE SOUND CLINICAL REASONING

To promote sound clinical reasoning, your assessments should have the following characteristics.

Purposeful. How you assess depends on your purpose and the circumstances (context) of your patient's situation. For example: Are you aiming to assess *all aspects* of care or *one specific problem?* Is your patient hospitalized or at home? Is the person an adult or a child? Always clarify your purpose and consider your patients' circumstances.

Prioritized. Be sure you gain the most important information *first*. There's certain information you should gain *early* because it's likely to affect virtually every aspect of care, including how you proceed with your assessment. We discuss this in detail later when we discuss *Quick Priority Assessments*.

Focused and Relevant. Focus your assessment to gain the relevant facts you need to completely understand your particular patient's problems, issues, and risks.

Systematic. Being systematic helps you to be comprehensive and to recognize if you have omitted something important.

Accurate and Complete. The most common error that happens in clinical reasoning is identifying problems or making judgments based on insufficient or incorrect data. Your information must be factual and as complete as is warranted by your purpose. For example, an assessment that aims to get information about *one specific problem* is shorter than one that aims to get comprehensive data about *all aspects of care*.

Recorded in a Standard Way. Recording information in a standard way ensures that the *most important information* can easily be found by all of the health care team, thereby promoting communication among caregivers.

SIX PHASES OF ASSESSMENT

The following six phases of *Assessment* help you gain the facts you need for the next step, *Diagnosis*.

1. **Collecting Data:** Gather information about health status.
2. **Identifying Cues and Making Inferences:** Identify cues (abnormal data) and draw some beginning conclusions about what the data may indicate.
3. **Validating (Verifying) Data:** Making sure that the data you gathered are factual and complete.
4. **Clustering Related Data:** Group related pieces of information together to help you to identify patterns of health or illness (e.g., clustering data about respiratory status together, data about nutrition status, and so forth).
5. **Identifying Patterns/Testing First Impressions:** Look for patterns and focus your assessment to gain more information to better understand the issues at hand. For example, you suspect that someone's data show a pattern of poor nutrition and decide to find out what's contributing to this pattern (does the person have poor eating habits or could it be something else, such as not having enough money to eat well?).
6. **Reporting and Recording Data:** Report abnormal data (e.g., a fever) and chart these on the patient's record according to policies and procedures.

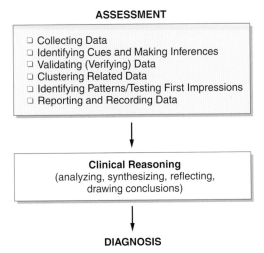

ASSESSMENT

- ❑ Collecting Data
- ❑ Identifying Cues and Making Inferences
- ❑ Validating (Verifying) Data
- ❑ Clustering Related Data
- ❑ Identifying Patterns/Testing First Impressions
- ❑ Reporting and Recording Data

Clinical Reasoning
(analyzing, synthesizing, reflecting,
drawing conclusions)

DIAGNOSIS

FIGURE 2.1   How the phases of *Assessment* set the stage for *Diagnosis.*

RULE   *Assessment* **is a** *process*—**the six phases addressed in this chapter are dynamic and interrelated.** For instance, *recording data* (part of the last phase) helps ensure that the first phase *(collecting data)* is accurate and complete: When you record the data, you often identify things you missed in your original assessment. Another example: *clustering related data* (phase 4) also helps you *validate the information* (phase 3) and make sure it's accurate and complete.

Figure 2.1 shows how the six phases of *Assessment* lead to *Diagnosis.*

COLLECTING DATA

Assessment begins with *collecting data*, an ongoing process that starts with patient admission and continues until discharge.

What Resources Do You Use?

The following summarizes the resources to use when gathering data.

- Patients and significant others
- Assessment technology (e.g., cardiac and respiratory monitors)
- Electronic and print health records
- Consultations with other experts (e.g., physicians, pharmacists, dieticians, clinical nurse specialists)
- Additional key stakeholders (e.g., caregivers, primary care providers, insurance companies)

Box 2.1	### Scenario: Assess Patients First—Then the Technology

Inexperienced nurses tend to believe all electronic information to be correct. However, remember that the patient is the primary source of information. For instance, imagine that you're looking after "Bob." He has a pulse oximeter—a device that's attached to his finger to measure blood oxygen saturation (called O2Sat). A normal O2Sat is 95%–100% (in some cases as low as 90% is acceptable). You assess Bob, and find that his O2Sat is 84. He has normal vital signs and no respiratory or cardiac symptoms. Do you believe the technology or your direct assessment of Bob? As the human in this interface with technology, check whether the pulse oximeter is correctly attached and working. On the other hand, if the O2Sat is normal, but Bob's lips are blue, he may be in trouble. To ensure valid assessment, consider BOTH the technology AND the patient—but, ASSESS PATIENTS FIRST.

RULE   **Always consider your *direct assessment of the patient* to be your primary source of information.**

Consider how the above rule applies to the scenario in Box 2.1.

Ensuring Comprehensive Data Collection

Comprehensive data collection occurs at three points in time.

1. **Before you see the patient:** You find out what you can. This information may be limited (only name and age) or extensive (you may have medical records to review).
2. **When you see the patient:** You interview the person and do a physical examination.
3. **After you see the patient:** You review the resources you used and determine what *other resources* may offer additional information (e.g., you may consult with a pharmacist to gain more information about a medication regimen).

DATA BASE, FOCUS, AND QUICK PRIORITY ASSESSMENTS

There are three main types of assessments:

1. **Data base (start of care) assessment:** Comprehensive information you gather on *initial contact* with the person to assess *all aspects* of health status.
2. **Focus assessment:** Information you gather to determine the status of a *specific* issue—for example, how a patient manages his diabetes.
3. **Quick Priority Assessments (QPAs):** These are short, focused, prioritized assessments that you do to gain the most important information you need to have *first*.

Data Base (Start of Care) Assessment

Data base (start of care) assessment tools are designed to ensure that the major information that's required to plan and give care is easily found (this is often called the minimum data set—the minimum that must be collected for every patient). Figure 2.2 shows a data base assessment tool. This tool is usually displayed in several computer screens.

**COMPLETE THIS SECTION FOR ALL PATIENTS
UNLESS SPECIFIC ASSESSMENT IS WARRANTED**

Patient Name: _____

CULTURE/RELIGIOUS/SPIRITUAL	ACTION TAKEN
Religious Preference: ☐ None ☐ Catholic ☐ Protestant ☐ Jewish ☐ Other _____ Any special cultural, spiritual, or religious needs while in the hospital? ☐ NO ☐ Yes Specify: _____	☐ Refer to Chaplain ☐ Other Referral
SOCIAL/DISCHARGE PLANNING	**ACTION TAKEN**
☐ Lives Alone ☐ Stairs ☐ Bathroom on same level as living quarters ☐ Lives with spouse/significant other/family/caretaker ☐ Lives in nursing home/assisted living ❶ ☐ Compromised in ADLs and/or lack of support network ❶ ☐ Special discharge needs ❶_____ ☐ Insurance concerns ❶ ☐ Received supports prior to admission: ☐ unknown ☐ home care ☐ med equip ❶ ☐ Patient plans to be discharged to: _____ ☐ Discharge Transportation (Name) _____ (Phone#) _____ ☐ Unable to return to pervious living arrangement ❷ ☐ Financial concerns ❷ ☐ Evidence of physical/emotional abuse or neglect or domestic violence ❷ ☐ Current substance abuse ❷ ☐ No discharge planning needs identified	☐ Assist With ADLs ☐ Patient Education ❶ ☐ Refer to Case Manager Referral ❷ ☐ Refer to Social Work Referral

EDUCATION NEEDS ASSESSMENT

Learning Readiness: ☐ Willing to Learn ☐ Unable to Learn
Barriers to Learning: ☐ No Barriers ☐ Cognitive ☐ Cultural ☐ Educational ☐ Emotional
 ☐ Language ☐ Motivational ☐ Financial ☐ Physical ☐ Religious ☐ Refuses at this time
 ☐ Comments/Other _____

Plans to Overcome Barriers to Education: ☐ Family involvement ☐ Reinforcement ☐ Written Materials
 ☐ Audiovisual Aids ☐ Interpreter ☐ Other _____

Special Educational Needs: ☐ Disease Process ☐ Activity Level ☐ Diet ☐ Procedures ☐ Hygiene
 ☐ Medications (including Drug and Food Interactions) ☐ Medical Equipment/Assistive Devices
 ☐ Skin/Ostomy (Certified wound Ostomy Continence notified)
 ☐ Other _____

Teaching to be directed primarily to: ☐ Patient ☐ Family ☐ Other _____
Patient Folder Given? ☐ Yes ☐ No

Clinical Pathway Initiated? ☐ Yes ☐ See Flowsheet/Progress Note

Correct ID band in place ☐ Yes
 ☐ Patient Handbook/Patient's Right and Responsibilities reviewed.
 ☐ Patient/family oriented to room

Completed by RN: _____ Date: _____ Time: _____

Reviewed by RN: _____ Date: _____ Time: _____

FIGURE 2.2 Data base admission tool; usually incorporated into several computer screens. (Reprinted with permission from Paoli Memorial Hospital, Paoli, Pennsylvania.)

Main Line Health

Jefferson Health System

☐ Paoli Hospital   ☐ Lankenau Hospital
☐ Bryn Mawr Hospital

INITIAL PATIENT ASSESSMENT

Complete shaded area **OR**   ☐ See 24 Hour Flow Sheet   ☐ See E.D. Triage Sheet
                                ☐ See Critical Care Pathway

Date:	Time:	Height:	Weight:	Language spoken other than English:

Primary Care Physician: _____   Specialist: _____

Vital Signs   Temp _____   P_____   RR_____   BP_____
              O2 Sat _____   O2 _____   RA _____

Reason for procedure/hospitalization: _____

Procedure: _____

Allergies: Drug/Food/Latex/Tape/Dyes   ☐ None Known

ALLERGIES	REACTION		ALLERGIES	REACTION		ALLERGIES	REACTION

ALL MEDICATIONS	☐ SENT HOME	☐ TO PHARMACY				
(Included over-the-counter drugs, vitamins, diet pills, and herbals currently being taken)	Dose	Route	Frequency	Last Taken	Reason for Taking/Comments
1.					
2.					
3.					
4.					
5.					
6.					
7.					
8.					
9.					
10.					
11.					

Recent Aspirin/Ibuprofen/Anti-inflammatory/Vitamin E/Blood Thinner: _____

PAST SURGICAL HISTORY

Past surgical History: _____

Previous anesthesia: ☐ General   ☐ Spinal   ☐ Other _____

Problems with Anesthesia? _____

Blood Donations-This Admission   ☐ Autologous   ☐ Direct Donor   ☐ None

FIGURE 2.2   *(Continued)*

Patient Name: _____   MR #: _____

HEALTH HISTORY	Check Applicable Boxes Only

NEUROLOGIC	CARDIOVASCULAR	RESPIRATORY	GASTROINTESTINAL
☐ CVA/TIA	☐ High Blood Pressure/	☐ Emphysema/Bronchitis	☐ Hiatal Hernia/Reflux
☐ Speech Difficulty	☐ Low Blood Pressure	☐ Asthma	☐ Hepatitis
☐ Swallowing/Choking	☐ Aneurysm	☐ Shortness of breath	☐ Ulcers
☐ Blackouts/Fainting/Vertigo	☐ Heart Attack	☐ TB	☐ Crohn's/Colitis
☐ Seizures	☐ Heart Failure	☐ Pneumonia	☐ Gall Bladder Disease
☐ Migraine/Headaches	☐ Murmur	☐ Seasonal/Environmental	☐ Irritable Bowels
☐ Numbness/Tingling	☐ Chest Pain/Angina	☐ Allergies	☐ Diverticular Disease
☐ Confusion	☐ Irregular Pulse	☐ Snoring/Apnea	☐ Ostomy _____
☐ Memory Changes	☐ Circulation Problem	☐ Breathing Devices: ____	☐ Recent change in bowel habits
☐ Head Injury	☐ Phlebitis/Clots		☐ Blood in stool
☐ Other _____	☐ Pacemaker/Defib.	☐ Other _____	☐ Last B.M. _____
☐ No identified problems	☐ High Cholesterol	No identified problems	☐ Other _____
	☐ Other _____		☐ No identified problems
	☐ No identified problems		

Comments: _____

MUSCULOSKELETAL	GENITOURINARY	PSYCHOSOCIAL	MISCELLANEOUS
☐ Arthritis	☐ Kidney Stones	☐ Alcohol use _____	☐ Vision Changes
☐ Muscle Weakness	☐ Prostate Problems	☐ Drug use _____	☐ Hearing Deficit
☐ Joint Replacement ____	☐ Ostomy	☐ Panic/Anxiety Attacks	☐ Glaucoma/Cataracts
☐ Spinal Problems	☐ Burning/Urgency Frequency	☐ Depression	☐ Blood/Bleeding Disorders
☐ Other _____	☐ Blood in Urine	☐ Physical/Psychological	☐ CA _____
☐ No identified problems	☐ Kidney Failure	☐ Abuse	☐ Skin Problems
METABOLIC	☐ Dialysis	☐ Tobacco use _____	☐ Hearing Deficit
☐ Diabetes Type: ____	☐ Breast Masses/	☐ Claustrophobia	☐ Infectious Disease/STD
☐ Thyroid	☐ Tenderness/Discharge	☐ ADD	☐ Head Circumference ____
☐ Hypoglycemia	☐ LMP _____	☐ Growth and Development	(if appropriate)
☐ Anemia	☐ Possibility of Pregnancy	not appropriate for age	☐ Immunizations up to date
☐ Other _____	☐ Breast Feeding	☐ Bereavement	(< > = 18 yrs)
☐ No identified problems	☐ Other _____	☐ Other _____	☐ Other _____
	☐ No identified problems	☐ No identified problems	☐ No identified problems

Comments: _____

Needs Assessment

☐ Orthodontic appliance	☐ Prosthesis	☐ Religious Items
☐ Dentures _____	☐ Glasses/Contacts	☐ Crutches/Walker/Cane/Wheelchair
☐ Hearing Aid	☐ Hairpiece	☐ Other _____

CURRENT PAIN		CARE OR LEARNING NEED

☐ Denies Pain		☐ Pain Management ☐ Patient Education
		Indicate in the diagram where
Duration of Pain? _____		pain is located and label the intensity 1-10, with "1" meaning
What Controls the Pain: ____		minimal pain to "10" being the worst pain
What is the Impact on ADLs?		

INTEGUMENTARY	
☐ Skin problems	☐ Rash
☐ Tattoos	☐ Pressure Ulcers
☐ Lower leg/foot wounds	☐ Ecchymosis
☐ Old scars	☐ No identified problems
☐ Dry skin	

X = Pain
O = Wound

Advance Directives	☐ NA (Patient < 18 years old)	☐ Unable to Assess

Does the patient have an advance directive?	☐ Yes	☐ No ☐ Information Given ☐ Information Declined
If "Yes" copy in current chart? Obtain from previous chart	☐ Yes	☐ No Follow-up action: ☐ Family to obtain copy for record ☐ Patient to formulate another advance directive (sample in "It's Up To You") ☐ Substance as stated by patient: _____
If "No" does the patient wish to make an advance directive?	☐ Yes-Refer to Social Work	☐ No ☐ Patient declines stated context ☐ Patient/family declines to bring, and/or complete advance directive information

FIGURE 2.2   (Continued)

COMPLETE THIS SECTION FOR INPATIENTS ONLY
UNLESS SPECIFIC ASSESSMENT IS WARRANTED

Patient Name: ————————————————————— MR #: ———————————

NUTRITIONAL STATUS	□ No Identified Problems	ACTION/TAKEN
If any of the following are present, send computer order to Nutrition Services □ Any Specific diet and/or restrictions ❶ □ Unintentional Weight Loss/Gain 10 lbs in the Last 6 Months ❶ □ Vomiting/Diarrhea for the Last 3 Days or Longer❶ □ Poor Appetite for the Last 5 Days or Longer ❶ □ Swallowing Difficulties resulting in inadequate intake❶ □ Newly Diagnosed Pt with Diabetes Need for Education❶, ❷ □ Pressure Ulcer Stage II or greater ❶, ❸ □ Dialysis ❶ □ New to modified Diet and Needs Education ❶		❶ □ Nutrition Referral ❷ □Diabetes Educator Referral ❸ □Certified Wound Ostomy Continence Nurse Referral

RESPIRATORY ASSESSMENT	□ No Identified Problems	ACTION/TAKEN
□ Patient is pre-op for upper abdominal or thoracic surgery and has a history of Emphysema, Bronchitis, Asthma, or Pulmonary Fibrosis		□ Respiratory Care Referred

FUNCTIONAL STATUS ASSESSMENT	□ No Identified Problems			ACTION/TAKEN
	Independent	Some Assist	Total Assist	□ Assist with ADL's
Feeding				
Bathing				
Dressing				
Toileting				
Transfer (bed to chair, to/from toilet)				
Walking/Use of Wheelchair				□Patient/Family Education

If any of the following are present, refer as follows:	□ Physician Order Requested
OCCUPATIONAL THERAPY □ No Needs Identified □ Condition Resulted in difficulty in use of one or both arms. □ Decreased Ability for Self-Care That Could Be Helped With Therapy. □ Physically Unable To Feed Self	For: OCCUPATIONAL THERAPY

PHYSICAL THERAPY   □ No Needs Identified
□ Condition has Resulted in Walking, and Transfer That Could Be
  Resolved with Therapy.
□ Condition has Resulted in Decreased Strength and/or Range of Motion
  of arms and legs.
□ Condition has Resulted in Acute Increase in Muscle or Back Pain.
	PHYSICAL THERAPY

SPEECH THERAPY □ No Needs Identified □ Difficulty Swallowing or Signs of Choking While Drinking/Eating. □ Diagnosis of Stroke, Myasthenia Gravis and Multiple Intubations. □ Unable to Follow Simple Instructions for Daily Care and/or Unable to Communicate Wants and Needs.	SPEECH/LANGUAGE PATHOLOGY

FALL RISK ASSESSMENT* Low Risk 0–20 Moderate Risk 25–60 High Risk 65–100 *See Patient Safety: Fall Safety Program		
Fall Assessment Indicators	**Weight Score**	**Assessment Score**
Admission or transfer	5	
History of falls	20	
Recent change in functional mobility	20	
Alteration in elimination	20	
Diagnosis/Medication which effects cognition/mobility/balance	10	
Confusion/impairment of judgment/forgetful/agitated and or non-compliant	20	
Sensory/Visual/Perceptual impairment (unrelated to above)	5	
TOTAL SCORE	100	

FIGURE 2.2   *(Continued)*

Focus Assessment

You may do a *focus assessment* as part of a data base assessment or by itself to monitor specific aspects of care. The following are the types of questions you need to ask during initial and ongoing focus assessments.

Examples of Initial Focus Assessment Questions

- What are your symptoms?
- Can you point with one finger to the areas that are bothering you?
- When did they start?
- What makes them better?
- What makes them worse?
- Are you taking any medications—prescribed, over-the-counter, or herbal remedies—that may be causing some of these symptoms?
- What else might be contributing to your symptoms?

Examples of Ongoing Focus Assessment Questions

- **What's the current status of the problem** (are there signs, symptoms, or risk factors for the problem)?
- **Compared with the baseline data** (data gathered before treatment began), does the information indicate that the problem is better, worse, or the same?
- **What factors are contributing to the problem,** and what has been done about these factors?
- **What's the patient's perspective** on the current status of the problem and how it's being managed?

Figure 2.3 (next page) shows a focus assessment tool for skin assessment. This tool is usually displayed on one or more computer screens. Figure 2.4 shows a computer screen from a focus assessment addressing fall risks.

Quick Priority Assessments (QPA)

Knowing how to do QPAs is important for two reasons:

1. These assessments "flag" existing problems and risks.
2. The information you gain often affects every aspect of care, including how you proceed with your assessment. For example, if your patient shows signs of a communicable disease, you need to immediately consider what precautions to take before going on with the rest of the assessment.

Box 2.2 on page 58 shows an example QPA.

FOCUS ASSESSMENT: SKIN

Note to the patient: Please help us assess your problem by taking a few moments to complete the self-assessment below. To give you the best care possible, we need you to pay attention to your body and keep us informed. In accordance with national safety goals, we want **YOU** to be a key player in all your health care decisions. Please speak up if you have any concerns.

Are you experiencing any of the below? (Use back of page if you need more room.)

	Yes	No	Where?	Started When?	What Makes it Better?	What Makes It Worse?
Itching						
Tingling						
Pain						
Swelling						
Redness						
Rash						
Blisters						
Drainage						
Lumps/ Lesions/ Moles						
Circulation Problems						

Other Important Questions To Think About...

	Yes	No
Have you been exposed to heat, direct sunlight, or tanning beds?		
Do you have any other symptoms, like fatigue or fever?		
Have you been exposed to chicken pox, measles, or anything like that?		
Have you been wearing clothes that fit tightly anywhere on your body?		
Are you taking any medications that have skin side effects? (List meds below)		
Anything else you want us to know? (Write on back of page)		

☐ **Any Allergies (include medications)?**

☐ **Medications (Include herbal and over-the-counter meds):**

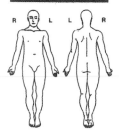

Mark Problems Below

FIGURE 2.3   Focus assessment tool; usually incorporated into electronic records.

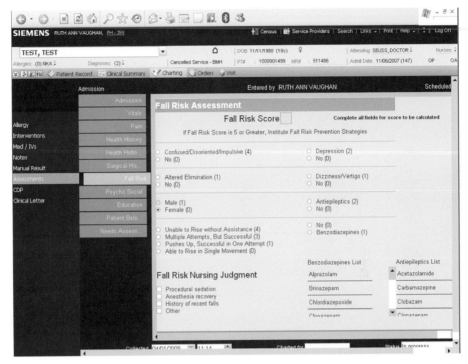

FIGURE 2.4   Computer screen showing focus assessment for risk for falls. (Reprinted with permission from Paoli Memorial Hospital, Paoli, Pennsylvania.)

Also remember the following rule.

RULE   **Medication reconciliation**—making sure that you have a complete and up-to-date list of medications being taken by the patient—is so important that it must be considered a part of comprehensive, focus, and quick priority assessments.

STANDARD TOOLS, EVIDENCE-BASED PRACTICE, AND ELECTRONIC HEALTH RECORDS

Completing electronic or print standard tools at various points in care is required by standards and regulatory agencies. These tools are an example of *applying evidence-based practice* (EBP). EBP brings together *the best of what we know from research* and *the best of what we know from clinical experts*. Standard tools ensure that the most important information is recorded and communicated in the best way. Whether you're admitting patients, transferring patients, or simply recording daily assessments, one of the first questions you should ask is: Is there a standard record that I need to complete? Getting these tools *early* helps you learn the most important things you need

Box 2.2   Quick Priority Assessment (QPA)

DEFINITION: A QPA includes the things that you should find out *first* in all patient encounters. You often do the QPA categories in rapid succession, or at the same time (not necessarily one before the other).

Assessment Priorities	Rationale
● Risks for infection, injury, or violence.	Keeping patients, yourself, and others safe is top priority. Address risks for patient infection or transmission of infection to others immediately (follow policies and procedures). Do the same for injury and violence risks.
● Problems (or risks for problems) with breathing, comfort, vital signs, or communication.	Problems and risks in these areas should be dealt with *early*. They also point to problems in *other areas* (e.g., pain usually flags a problem that needs to be dealt with).
● Allergies ● Current medications and treatments ● Admitting Diagnosis/Chief Complaint ● Current and past medical problems ● Current and past nursing problems.	These flag known problems and risks and affect decisions about initiating certain treatments.

Source: © 2011. www.AlfaroTeachSmart.com.

to assess in each particular situation. Figure 2.5 (next page) shows the SBAR tool, a common standard tool that's used to improve nurse-to-nurse and nurse-to-physician communication.

RULE   Electronic health records (EHR), Health Information Technology (HIT), and other standard tools promote sound clinical reasoning, but they don't think *for* you.

Just as pilots use Federal Aviation Administration–approved tools to reduce errors at various points in flight, you'll be required to use approved tools at specific points during patient care (e.g., when you admit or transfer patients). These tools help you be systematic and comprehensive. But they don't *think* for you. YOU are the one who has to do the critical thinking needed to ensure that the *information you record on the tools* is factual, relevant, and complete. YOU are the one who has to develop *assessment habits* that help you make clinical decisions. YOU are the one who has to have these habits "in your head" to be able to pass NCLEX and other tests.

SBAR (Situation, Background, Assessment, Recommendation)*

NOTE: Pronounced S-BAR and first used by the military to improve the effectiveness of communication between care givers, the SBAR approach is recommended by patient safety experts. SBAR forms vary depending on purpose and setting. Some places use SBAR for giving hand-off situations (when one nurse transfers patient care to another). Some places use SBAR forms like the one below for calling physicians about a problem.

→ Have the chart in hand before you make the phone call, and be sure you can readily communicate all of the following information.

S SITUATION: Have the chart in hand before you make the phone call, and be sure you can readily communicate all the following: Briefly state the issue or problem: what it is, when it happened (or how it started) and how severe it is. Give the signs and symptoms that cause you concern.

B BACKGROUND: Give the date of admission and current medical diagnoses. Determine the pertinent medical history and give a brief synopsis of the treatment to date (e.g., medications; oxygen use; nasogastric tube; IVs, code status).

A ASSESSMENT: Give most recent vital signs and any changes in the following:

- ☐ Mental status – neuro signs
- ☐ Respirations
- ☐ Pulse – skin color
- ☐ Comfort – Pain
- ☐ GI status (nausea-vomiting-diarrhea, distention)
- ☐ Urine Output
- ☐ Bleeding-Drainage
- ☐ Other: _____

R RECOMMENDATION: State what you think should be done. For example:

- ☐ Come see the patient now
- ☐ Get a consultation
- ☐ Get additional studies (e.g., CXR, ABG, EKG, CBC, other)
- ☐ Transfer the patient to ICU
- ☐ If the patient doesn't improve
- ☐ How frequent do you want vital signs.
- ☐ If there's no improvement, by when do you want us to call you?

*Data from: Haig, K, Sutton, S. and Whittington, J. (2006) SBAR: A Shared Mental Model for Improving Communication Between Clinicians. *Journal of Quality and Patient Safety*, 32(3), 167–175.
Source: R. Alfaro-LeFevre Handouts © 2007-2008 www.AlfaroTeachSmart.com

FIGURE 2.5   SBAR Tool promotes consistent communication.

ASSESSING DISEASE AND DISABILITY MANAGEMENT

Many patients today live with chronic conditions—for example, diabetes, asthma, heart disease, cancer, or paralysis. You need to assess these conditions *early* for the following reasons:

1. **You must be sure that the medical plan is current.** You're responsible for ensuring that all medical problems are being managed by a qualified primary care provider.

2. **How you manage nursing care is influenced by the medical treatment plan.** (e.g., if you decide you need to encourage fluids in a patient with heart disease, you need to know whether the physician has prescribed fluid restrictions).

3. **You need to find out how patients manage their diseases or disabilities, as this will also influence nursing care.** Patients are the experts on how they manage their own care. If they're managing their diseases and disabilities well, follow their plan as much as possible (don't assume you have a better way). If they're managing these poorly, find out *why* so that the reasons can be addressed in the plan of care (e.g., is there a lack of knowledge or is the problem a lack of resources?).

4. **You're responsible for ensuring that patients have the knowledge and skills to manage their own health problems.** (see Patient Education—Empowering Patients and Families in Chapter 4).

HEALTH PROMOTION: SCREENING FOR RISK MANAGEMENT AND EARLY DIAGNOSIS

Increasingly today, your assessments will include screening for risk management and early diagnosis of common health problems. Screening is often done at significant points during the life cycle. For example:

- Assessing infant development
- Measuring height, weight, and vision in school-age children
- Assessing for depression and drug and alcohol abuse, beginning in adolescence
- Measuring cholesterol and fecal blood in adults

You may be also be required to do specific health promotion counseling (e.g., smoking cessation) during all important interactions.

Partnering With Patients to Make Informed Decisions

As we realize the importance of patient-centered care, we also realize the importance of partnering with patients to make informed decisions about what screening and prevention measures they should follow. This means moving from a *paternalistic* model ("we know what's best for you") to a *partnership* model ("we want you to be informed so that you can *choose the best for you*"). The following summarizes information from U.S. Preventive Services Task Force (USPSTF) related to discussing health screening with patients[2]:

The length of discussions about screening for health problems and use of medication to prevent diseases varies according to:

- The scientific evidence addressing how useful the service is
- The health, preferences, and concerns of each patient
- The decision-making style of each clinician
- Practical constraints, such as the amount of time available

The USPSTF points out that you can consider your patients decisions to be informed and mutually decided only if they:

- Understand the risks or seriousness of the disease or condition to be prevented
- Comprehend what the preventive service involves (including the risks, benefits, alternatives, and uncertainties)
- Have weighed their values about the potential benefits and harm associated with the service
- Have engaged in decision making at a level at which they want and feel comfortable

ETHICAL, CULTURAL, AND SPIRITUAL CONCERNS

The success of your assessments is influenced by your awareness of ethical, cultural, and spiritual concerns.[1,3] According to professional standards, it's your responsibility to:

1. **Assess with respect for human dignity** and the uniqueness of the patient, unrestricted by considerations of social or economic status, personal attributes, or the nature of health problems.
2. **Safeguard the client's right to privacy** by judiciously protecting information of a confidential nature. This is also law.
3. **Be honest.** Tell the person the truth about how you'll use the data (e.g., "I have to write a paper examining someone's eating patterns. Would you be willing to tell me about your eating habits?").
4. **Respect cultural and religious beliefs** and be aware of physical tendencies related to culture. This includes being aware of:
   - **Biologic variations.** For example, differences among racial and ethnic groups (e.g., skin color and texture, and susceptibility to diseases like hypertension or sickle cell anemia).
   - **Comfortable communication patterns.** For example, how language and gestures are used, whether eye contact or touching is acceptable, and whether the person is threatened by being in close proximity to another.
   - **Family organization and practices.** We have diverse family units and practices. We must understand them to gain insight into factors that influence health status.
   - **Beliefs about whether people are able to control nature and influence their ability to be healthy** (e.g., whether blood transfusions are allowed or whether rituals are required).
   - **The person's concept of "God" and beliefs about the relationship between spiritual beliefs and health status** (e.g., "God gives you what you deserve.").

THE INTERVIEW AND PHYSICAL ASSESSMENT

The nursing interview and physical assessment complement and clarify each other, as you can see in the following example.

EXAMPLE

You interview a woman who tells you, "My breathing doesn't feel right." You take a stethoscope and listen to her lungs. What you hear (whether the breath sounds are normal or abnormal) gives you additional information that complements and clarifies what you've been told.

Developing Your Interviewing Skills

Interpersonal and communication skills—your ability to *establish rapport, ask questions, listen, and observe*—are central to building a therapeutic relationship and performing an assessment. People seeking health care are in an extremely vulnerable position, as they have few choices. It's your job to help people feel like they're in good hands and that their main concerns will be addressed.

Guidelines: Promoting a Caring Interview

The following can help you to establish trust, create a positive attitude, and reduce anxiety

How to Establish Rapport

Before You Go Into the Interview

- **Get organized.** Be sure you have everything you need to have with you.
- **Don't rely on memory:** Have a printed or electronic assessment tool to guide the questions you'll ask (e.g., use a standard tool).
- **Plan enough time:** The admission interview usually takes 30–60 minutes.
- **Ensure privacy:** Make sure you have a quiet, private setting, free from interruptions or distractions.
- **Get focused:** Clear your mind of other concerns (other duties, worries about yourself). Say to yourself, "Getting to know this person is the most important thing I have to do right now."
- **Visualize yourself as being confident, warm, and helpful:** This helps you to *be* confident, warm, and helpful—your genuine interest comes through.

When You Begin the Interview

- **Introduce yourself and give your name and position.** This sends the message that you accept responsibility and are willing to be accountable for your actions. This is especially important if you are a student.

- **Verify the person's name and ask what he or she would like to be called** (e.g., "I have your name as Jack Riley. Is that correct? What would you like us to call you?"). Use the preferred name to help the person feel more relaxed and send the message that you recognize that this person is an individual who has likes and dislikes.

RULE In accordance with national patient safety goals, use at least two unique identifiers to be sure you have the right patient.[4] For example, ask the person his name and birth date and also check the ID bracelet to make sure it matches what he says.

- **Briefly explain your purpose** (e.g., "I'm here to do the admission interview to help us plan your nursing care.").

During the Interview

- **Give the person your full attention.** Avoid the impulse to become engrossed in your notes or computer.
- **Avoid rushing.** It sends the message that you're not interested in what the person has to say.

How to Listen

- **Listen actively—listen for feelings as well as words.** Someone who sighs, looks away, and says, "I'll be okay with this," might be telling you, "I doubt this will work."
- **Let the person know when you see body language that sends a message that conflicts with what is being said** (e.g., "You say that you aren't having pain, but you look uncomfortable to me.").
- **Use short, supplementary phrases that let the person know you understand** and encourage the person to continue. Some examples are, "I see," "Mm-hm," "Oh, no," "And...," and "Then what?" A nod of the head and maintaining eye contact also lets the person know that you're listening.
- **Be patient if the person has a memory block.** This information may be remembered later when you ask related questions.
- **Avoid the impulse to interrupt.** If the interview is getting off track, allow people to finish sentences, then say, "We're getting off track. Can we get back to...?"
- **Allow for pauses in conversation.** Silence gives both you and the person time to gather thoughts, and allows you to reflect on the accuracy of the information the patient has provided.

How to Ask Questions

- **Ask about the person's main problems first** (e.g., "What are the main reasons you're here today?").
- **Focus your questions to gain specific information about signs and symptoms.** (e.g., "Show me where the problem is." "Can you describe how this feels

more specifically?" "When did this start?" "When does this seem to happen?" "Is there anything that makes it better?" "What makes it worse?")

● **Don't use leading questions** (questions that lead the person to a specific response; e.g., "You don't smoke, do you?" leads the person to a "no" answer).
● **Do use exploratory statements** (statements that begin with words like tell, describe, explain, and elaborate) to get the person to tell you more about specific conditions (e.g., "Tell me more about your sleeping patterns."). Some authors use the term *leading statements* instead of *exploratory statements*. I use *exploratory statements* to avoid confusion with *leading questions*, which you *should not* use.
● **Use communication techniques that enhance your ability to think critically and get the facts:**
    1. **Use phrases that help you see the other person's perspective** (e.g., "From your point of view, what are the biggest problems?" or "What are the problems as you see them?").
    2. **Restate the person's own words.** This technique clarifies meaning and encourages the person to expand on what's been said (e.g., "When you say..., what do you mean?" or "When you say..., does this mean... ?" or "Let me repeat what you said to make sure I understand.").
    3. **Ask open-ended questions** (questions requiring more than a one-word answer, such as "How are you feeling?" rather than "Are you feeling well?").
    4. **Avoid closed-ended questions** (those requiring a one-word answer) unless the person is too ill to elaborate or you're trying to clarify a response by getting a yes or no answer.

Table 2.1 gives examples of open-ended and closed-ended questions. Table 2.2 summarizes the advantages and disadvantages of using each of these types of questions.

What to Observe

● **Carefully assess areas connected to verbal complaints** (e.g., if someone has abdominal discomfort, focus your assessment carefully on the abdomen).
● **Use your senses.** Do you see, hear, or smell anything unusual?
● **Note general appearance.** Does the person appear well-groomed, healthy, well-nourished?

Table 2.1   Examples of Closed-Ended and Open-Ended Questions

Closed-Ended	Open-Ended
Are you happy about this?	How does this make you feel?
Do you get along with your husband?	How is your relationship with your husband?
Does this make you sick to your stomach?	How does this affect your stomach?

Table 2.2   Advantages and Disadvantages of Open-Ended and Closed-Ended Questions

Advantages	Disadvantages
Open-Ended Question	
Brings forth more information than a question that requires only a one-word response. Gives people a chance to verbalize and involves them in dialogue. Tends to bring forth a more honest reply. Usually less threatening and less likely to convey negative judgment. Often interpreted to imply sincere interest.	May allow the person to sidestep the question. Requires a more wordy response. This may be undesirable in an emergency situation or if the individual is confused, in pain, or having difficulty breathing. Allows opportunity to ramble and get off track.
Closed-Ended Question	
Helps clarify responses to open-ended questions. Saves time in emergency situations. Can be helpful in focusing the interview on specific data (e.g., following a checklist that asks for history of specific illnesses, such as high blood pressure, heart attacks). May be helpful for those who are confused, in pain, or having difficulty breathing.	May be more threatening. Limits the amount of information offered. Does not encourage the person to express concerns from his or her point of view. Does not encourage active dialogue between the nurse and the person.

- **Observe body language.** Does the person appear comfortable? Nervous? Withdrawn? Apprehensive? What behaviors do you see?
- **Notice interaction patterns.** Be aware of the person's responses to your interviewing style (e.g., sometimes cultural and personal differences create communication barriers).

How to Terminate the Interview

- **Give a warning** (e.g., "We have 5 minutes to finish up... let's be sure we have covered the most important things you want us to know.")
- **Ask people to summarize their most important concerns** and then summarize the most important concerns as you see them (e.g., "We've talked about a lot of things. To make sure I have it right, tell me the three most important things I can help you with.")
- **Ask, "what else?"** (e.g., "Is there anything else you want me to know?")
- **Offer yourself as a resource** (e.g., "I want to be kept informed on how you're doing. Let me know if something changes or if you have any questions.")
- **Explain care routines and provide information about who is accountable for nursing care decisions.** Patients are often confused about who is responsible for what.
- **End on a positive note and encourage the person to become an active participant.** (e.g., "We have a good start here. We want you to be actively involved in making decisions about your care.")

| Box 2.3 | **Avoid These Communication Errors** |

- **Using first names without permission** (it's disrespectful).
- **Using *honey, dear, sweetie, pop, or grandma.***
- **"Talking down."** For example, "So you've had a pain in your tummy?"
- **Using medical terminology with laypeople.** Many people don't know common medical terms such as void, vital signs, BM.
- **Ignoring patients' non-verbal communication.** For example, touching someone to offer support and not noticing that he withdraws, sending the message that he doesn't want to be touched.

Box 2.3 lists common communication errors to avoid.

Developing Your Physical Assessment Skills

Developing your physical assessment skills requires becoming systematic, thorough, and skilled in the following techniques.

- **Inspection:** Observing carefully by using your fingers, eyes, ears, and sense of smell
- **Auscultation:** Listening with a stethoscope
- **Palpation:** Touching and pressing to test for pain and feel inner structures, such as the liver
- **Percussion:** Directly or indirectly tapping a body surface to determine reflexes (done with a percussion hammer) or to determine whether an area contains fluid (done by tapping fingers over surface)

How you organize your assessment is influenced by three things:

1. **The person's condition:** If the person is ill or has a specific complaint, begin by examining the problem areas before going on to other parts of the body (e.g., if there's abdominal pain, examine the abdomen first; if someone is unconscious, assess neurological, respiratory, and cardiovascular status first).
2. **The standard tool or record that you're required to complete.** Often, these guide your approach.
3. **Your own preference.** You may choose a head-to-toe approach, beginning by assessing the head and neck, and continuing down the body to the thorax, abdomen, legs, and feet, in that order. Or you may choose a body systems approach such as the one in Box 2.4.

Guidelines: Performing a Physical Assessment

The following guidelines help you to develop habits that promote a thorough and systematic physical assessment.

Box 2.4	Systematic Head-to-Toe Physical Assessment

- **Neurologic status.** Check: mental status; orientation; pupil reaction; vision and appearance of the eyes; gag reflex; ability to hear, taste, feel, and smell; gait; coordination; arm and leg reflexes; presence of pain or discomfort (e.g., headache)
- **Respiratory status.** Check: throat, airway, breath sounds, rate and depth of breathing, cough, symmetry of chest expansion, presence of pain/discomfort (e.g., chest pain)
- **Cardiac and circulatory status.** Check: apical heart rate, rhythm, heart sounds; quality of pulses (radial, brachial, carotid, femoral, dorsalis pedis); presence of peripheral edema; presence of pain/discomfort (e.g., chest or extremity pain)
- **Skin status.** Check: color, temperature, skin turgor, edema, lesions, rashes, lumps, hair distribution. Specifically examine male and female breasts for lumps or nipple discharge. Check for itching/pain/discomfort.
- **Musculoskeletal status.** Check: muscle tone, strength, range of motion, presence of pain/discomfort (e.g., aches, spasm)
- **Gastrointestinal status.** Check: condition of the lips, tongue, gums, teeth; bowel sounds; presence of abdominal distention; impaction; hemorrhoids; presence of pain/discomfort (e.g., abdominal tenderness). If vomiting, check emesis for color and blood.
- **Genitourinary status.** Check color and amount of urine; presence of distended bladder; discharge (vaginal, urethral); condition of the vulva; testicular examination; presence of pain/discomfort

- **Promote communication.** Establish rapport, and use good interviewing techniques (rather than working in silence).
- **Provide privacy.** Uncover only the body parts being examined, keeping the rest of the body draped. Tell the person before touching a part of the body that she can't see (e.g., "I'm going to feel this cyst on your back.").
- **Don't rely on memory.** Jot down notes or enter the data directly into the compute.
- **Choose a way to organize your assessment and use it consistently, so that it becomes a habit.**

RULE	**Pain and cough are the "fifth and sixth" vital signs.** When taking

routine vital signs (temperature, pulse, respirations, and blood pressure), ask about the "fifth vital sign" (whether the person has pain or discomfort) and assess closely to determine the cause. Cough is the sixth vital sign. While complete lung assessment is important, you can learn a lot from brief encounters. You can say something like, "Can you cough for me so I can hear how it sounds?" The person's ability (or inability) to comply with this request tells you a lot—for example, whether the person has pain with coughing, whether there's congestion, or whether the person's cough effort is strong enough to clear the lungs.

This brief encounter can help you "flag" patients who need more in-depth assessment. (In some facilities, pulse oximetry is considered the sixth vital sign. Pulse oximetry is a non-invasive way to monitor the percentage of hemoglobin that is saturated with oxygen. The pulse oximeter consists of a probe attached to the patient's finger or ear lobe that is linked to an electronic unit).

Checking Diagnostic Studies

Your assessment is incomplete until you check results of diagnostic studies. These studies are like a "report card" on how the body is functioning—they provide key evidence that helps you to determine health status. The data you gathered during the interview and examination may be perfectly normal, but you could miss the serious problems if you don't check the lab studies (e.g., kidney, liver, and hematological problems are often silent). Diagnostic studies may also confirm your suspicions (e.g., you may suspect an infection and be able to confirm it by blood work).

CRITICAL THINKING AND CLINICAL REASONING EXERCISES

2.1

Developing Your Interview and Physical Assessment Skills

Example responses are provided at the end of the book (page 204).

Part One: Developing Your Interviewing Skills

1. **Practice asking open-ended questions.** Restate each of the following questions as an open-ended question.

   a. "Are you feeling better?"

   b. "Did you like dinner?"

   c. "Are you happy here?"

   d. "Are you having pain?"

2. **Practice clarifying communication by using reflective statements** (restating what you hear) and making open-ended questions. For each of the following statements, write a reflective statement and an open-ended question that would help you to clarify what has been said.

   a. "I've been sick off and on for a month."

   b. "Nothing ever goes right for me."

   c. "I seem to have a pain in my side that comes and goes."

   d. "I've had this funny feeling for a week."

3. **Test your knowledge of communication techniques.** Read each of the following sentences and identify whether it is an open-ended statement (O), a closed-ended statement (C), a leading question (L), an exploratory statement (E), or a supplementary phrase or statement intended to help the person continue (S).

   a. "Are you afraid of dying?"

   b. "Tell me when this first started."

   c. "I see."

   d. "You're not still afraid to feed Hector, are you?"

   e. "How do you think you'll be doing this at home?"

   f. "Do you have a history of hypertension in your family?"

   g. "And... ?"

   h. "You do want your family to visit, don't you?"

   i. "How do you feel about being here?"

   j. "You don't need more practice, do you?"

   k. "Explain what you mean by 'a long time.'"

4. **Rephrase each leading question that you identified in number 3** to an open-ended question.

Part Two: Developing Your Physical Assessment Skills

1. **Because physical assessment and interviewing go hand-in-hand,** use the following situations to practice focusing your interview questions on areas of concern noted during the physical examination.

   a. You examine and find: The patient's hands and fingernails are filthy with ground-in dirt, although the rest of him is clean. What will you say or ask next?

   b. You examine and find: The patient has a lump on the back of his head. What will you say or ask next?

   c. You examine and find: The patient's respirations are 40. What will you say or ask next?

   d. You examine and find: The patient's right eye is red, teary, and inflamed. What will you say or ask next?

2. **Practice focusing your physical examination on areas of concern voiced by the patient.**

   a. The patient states: "I have had a rash that comes and goes." What will you reply and examine?

   b. The patient states: "My stomach has been hurting me." What will you reply and examine?

   c. The patient states: "I find it burns when I urinate." What will you reply and examine?

   d. The patient states: "I feel like I'm heavier than usual, like I'm bloated with fluid." What will you reply and examine?

3. **Your approach to the interview and physical assessment** should be influenced by which of the following?

   a. Your own preference

   b. The patient's condition

   c. Both of the above

   d. Neither of the above

Try This on Your Own

1. Practice combining interviewing techniques with a physical examination. Do a mock interview and physical examination on a peer, friend, or family member using an assessment tool from school or a local clinical facility. Be sure you can explain *why* the form requires you to collect each piece of data because understanding why helps you learn the critical thinking skill of determining what's relevant.

2. Practice doing a focus assessment. Ask someone you know who is taking medications to allow you to do an assessment of their medication regimen. Use the following memory-jog TACIT to guide your assessment.

Using TACIT Memory-Jog to Assess Medication Regimens

T–Therapeutic effect? (Is there a therapeutic effect?)
A–Allergic or Adverse reactions? (Signs of allergic or adverse reactions?)
C–Contraindications? (Are there contraindications to giving this drug?)
I–Interactions? (Possible drug interactions?)
T–Toxicity/overdose? (Are there signs of toxicity or overdose?)

3. Discuss how doing a quick priority assessment (QPA) helps you prioritize your thinking during assessment (see example QPA in Box 2.2).

4. Learn more about health screening and prevention of common diseases at the following Web sites.
   - Agency For Healthcare Research and Quality (www.ahrq.gov/)
   - Healthy People (www.healthypeople.gov). Here you can download The *Guide to Clinical Preventive Services* includes USPSTF recommendations on screening, counseling, and preventive medication topics and including clinical considerations for each topic.
   - The Centers for Disease Control and Prevention Web page (www.cdc.gov/)
   - Harvard Center For Risk Analysis (www.hcra.harvard.edu/)

5. In a personal journal, with a peer, or in a group, discuss the implications of the following Voices and Think About It entries.

Voices

Communication, Cultural Competence, and Patient- and Family-Centered Care

"Patients have specific characteristics and nonclinical needs that can affect the way they view, receive, and participate in healthcare....research documents that a variety of patient populations experience decreased patient safety, poorer outcomes, and lower quality care based on race, ethnicity, language, disability, and sexual orientation. As cultural, communication, mobility, and other basic needs go unmet, hospitals will continue to put themselves and their patients at risk for negative consequences. To improve the overall safety and quality of care provided in hospitals nationwide, health care organizations should aspire to meet the unique needs of their patients—patient by patient."[5]

—The Joint Commission

Are You Seduced by Technology?

"Technology is at the heart of critical care. It allows clinicians to perform miracles, but is also a seductive and self-perpetuating force that needs careful monitoring by those who use it."[6]

—Marjorie Funk, PhD, RN, FAHA, FAAN

IDENTIFYING SUBJECTIVE AND OBJECTIVE DATA

Considering both *subjective data* (what the person states) and *objective data* (what you observe) aids clinical reasoning because each of these complements and clarifies the other. For example, notice how the following subjective data are supported by the objective data.

- **Subjective data:** States, "I feel like my heart is racing."
- **Objective data:** Right radial pulse 150 beats per minute, regular, and strong Sometimes, what you *observe* and what the person *states* are conflicting, as in the following data.
- **Subjective data: States, "I feel fine."**
- **Objective data:** Color pale, easily becomes short of breath

When you have conflicting subjective and objective data, you need to investigate more to understand the problems completely.

Use the following to remember the difference between these two terms:

S—S (Subjective data = Stated)
O—O (Objective data = Observed)

When you address subjective data, use the patients' *own words* (e.g., states "the pain comes and goes for no reason"). When you address objective data, use *specific, measurable terms* (e.g., *temperature of 100.6°F* is more specific and measurable than *temperature elevated*). The following gives examples of subjective and objective data.

EXAMPLE

Subjective Data	Objective Data
"I feel sick to my stomach."	Abdomen hard and distended
"My foot hurts."	Limps on left foot
"It burns when I urinate."	Urinated 150 mL clear urine

IDENTIFYING CUES AND MAKING INFERENCES

The subjective and objective data you identify act as *cues*. Cues are data that prompt you to get a beginning impression of patterns of health or illness. For example, consider the following cues.

- **Subjective data:** "I just started taking penicillin for a tooth abscess."
- **Objective data:** Fine rash over trunk

The above gives you cues that may lead you to infer (suspect) that there's an allergic reaction to penicillin. How you interpret or perceive a cue—the conclusion you draw about the cue—is called an *inference*.

Your ability to identify cues and make correct inferences is influenced by your observational skills, your nursing knowledge, and your clinical expertise. Your values and beliefs also affect how you interpret some cues; make an effort to avoid making value judgments (e.g., inferring that a person who bathes only once a week needs to be taught better hygiene, rather than wondering whether this could be a part of the person's culture).

To clarify your understanding of cues and inferences, study the following examples of cues and corresponding inferences.

EXAMPLE

Cue	Corresponding Inference
"I have trouble moving my bowels."	May be constipated.
"I don't want to talk."	May be depressed or angry.
Blood pressure 60/50.	Is in shock.
"I can't stand this pain anymore."	Has severe pain.

VALIDATING (VERIFYING) DATA

Validating (verifying) that your information is factual and complete is a crucial step in clinical reasoning. It helps you to avoid making the following mistakes:

- Making assumptions
- Missing key information

- Misunderstanding situations
- Jumping to conclusions or focusing in the wrong direction
- Making errors in problem identification

For instance, suppose you ask a woman whether she is pregnant, and she responds, "No." If you don't verify this by getting more information—for example, asking "When was your last menstrual period?" or finding out the results of a pregnancy test—you may proceed under the woman isn't pregnant when indeed she is. This can be dangerous, especially considering that drugs that may harm the fetus could be prescribed.

RULE Recognizing assumptions—recognizing when information has been taken for granted without being verified—is a key clinical reasoning skill. As humans, we're all vulnerable to making assumptions, especially when we're in new situations. Validating data—ensuring that the information you gathered is factual and complete—helps you uncover assumptions and make corrections early. Patient status is constantly changing. Remember: Check, check, and check again—the more you look, the more you find.

Guidelines: Validating (Verifying) Data

The following guidelines help you know how to ensure that your data are factual and complete.

- **Data that can be measured accurately can be accepted as being valid** (e.g., height, weight, diagnostic study results). However, keep in mind that there's always the possibility of a lab error or other factors that may alter the accuracy of studies (e.g., a fasting blood sugar test that's done even though the person ate an hour earlier).
- **Data that someone else observes (indirect data) may or may not be true. Verify** information by directly observing and interviewing the patient *yourself*.
- **The following techniques help you validate data.**
  - Double-check information that's extremely abnormal or inconsistent with patient cues (e.g., use two scales to check an infant who appears much heavier or lighter than the scale states; repeat an extremely high or low laboratory result).
  - Double-check that your equipment is working correctly.
  - Recheck your own data (e.g., take a patient's blood pressure in the opposite arm or 10 minutes later).
  - Look for factors that may alter accuracy (e.g., check whether someone who has an elevated temperature and no other symptoms has just had a hot cup of tea).
  - Ask someone else, preferably an expert, to collect the same data (e.g., ask a more experienced nurse to recheck a blood pressure when you're not sure).

- Compare subjective and objective data to see if what the person *states* is consistent with what you *observe* (e.g., compare actual pulse rate with perceptions of "racing heart").
- Verify your inferences with the patient (e.g., "You look uncomfortable.").
- Compare your impressions with those of other key members of the health care team (e.g., "He seems anxious.").
- When making decisions about whether data are valid or not, let the following rule play in your head.

RULE **More than one cue, more likely it's true—more than one source, more likely of course.** Clinical reasoning requires making judgments based on *evidence*. Look for *more than one cue* to support your conclusions. For example, if your patient's agitation causes you to suspect that there's a risk for violence, ask the family and check the chart for history of violence.

CRITICAL THINKING AND CLINICAL REASONING EXERCISES

2.2 Subjective and Objective Data; Cues and Inferences; Validating Data

Example responses are provided at the end of the book (pages 204–205).

Part One: Subjective and Objective Data

1. List the *subjective data* noted in the following case history that follows (what does Mr. Michaels *state?*).

   Case History

   Mr. Michaels gives his age as being 51 years old. He was admitted yesterday with chest pain. His physician has ordered the following studies: electrocardiogram, chest x-ray examination, and complete blood studies including a blood sugar test. Results of these studies were just posted on the chart. When you talk with Mr. Michaels, he states, "I feel much better today—no more pain. It is a relief to get rid of that discomfort." You think he appears a little tired or weary; he seems to be talking slowly and sighs more often than you think is normal. He denies being weary. His vital signs are as follows:
   T: 98.6   P: 74 (regular)   R: 22   BP: 140/90

2. List the *objective data* noted in the preceding case history (what information is *observed?*).

Part Two: Cues and Inferences

1. List the cues in the case history in Part One.

2. List the inferences that you might make about the cues you identified.

Part Three: Validating Data

1. Decide how valid the cues and inferences that you identified in Part Two are.

2. Identify some ways you could validate your cures and inferences.

Try This on Your Own

In a personal journal, with a peer, or in a group, discuss the implications of the following.

 ## Think About It

Trust, But Verify

"Trust, but verify" is an old Russian proverb that stresses the need to verify information, even when you believe the source. This proverb applies to keeping patients safe. Even when you've been given information that seems to be true, verify it as best you can.

CLUSTERING RELATED DATA

Just as putting similar puzzle pieces together helps you get a beginning idea of what the puzzle will look like when it's finished, clustering related health data together helps you get a beginning picture of various aspects of health status.

Assessment tools guide you to cluster data together (e.g., information about nutrition is mostly in one place, information about activity is mostly in one place, and so on). However, no tool does *all the clustering* you need to do to understand each and every problem. You have to *think* about the relationships among data on the tool. For example, the data clustered under *nutrition* also relate to data under *skin status* (poor nutrition is a risk factor for skin problems). The following section helps you to learn principles of clustering data that are central to clinical reasoning.

Box 2.5   Gordon's Functional Health Patterns

- **Health-Perception–Health-Management:** Perception of general health status and well-being. Adherence to preventive health practices.
- **Nutritional–Metabolic:** Patterns of food and fluid intake, fluid and electrolyte balance, general ability to heal.
- **Elimination:** Patterns of excretory function (bowel, bladder, and skin), and client's perception.
- **Activity–Exercise:** Pattern of exercise, activity, leisure, recreation, and activities of daily living; factors that interfere with desired or expected individual pattern.
- **Cognitive–Perceptual:** Adequacy of sensory modes, such as vision, hearing, taste, touch, smell, pain perception, cognitive functional abilities.
- **Sleep–Rest:** Patterns of sleep and rest/relaxation periods during 24-hour day, as well as quality and quantity.
- **Self-Perception–Self-Concept:** Attitudes about self, perception of abilities, body image, identity, general sense of worth, and emotional patterns.
- **Role–Relationship:** Perception of major roles and responsibilities in current life situation.
- **Sexuality–Reproductive:** Perceived satisfaction or dissatisfaction with sexuality. Reproductive stage and pattern.
- **Coping–Stress-Tolerance:** General coping pattern, stress tolerance, support systems, and perceived ability to control and manage situations.
- **Value–Belief:** Values, goals, or beliefs that guide choices or decisions.

Source: Summarized from Gordon, M. (2011). *Manual of nursing diagnosis* (12th ed). Burlington, MA: Jones & Bartlett Learning.

Clustering Data According to Your Purpose

Many nurses want *one way* to cluster data to meet all purposes. However, remember "one size doesn't fit all" and "more than one way is a must today." If you cluster data only one way, you get a narrow view and may miss important problems. You have to be sure that you cluster your data according to your purpose. For example, clustering data according to *Gordon's Functional Health Patterns* (Box 2.5) helps you identify nursing concerns, but it isn't very helpful for setting priorities—*Maslow's Hierarchy of Human Needs* (Box 2.6) is better for this purpose.

Figure 2.6 shows the relationship between clustering data and identifying health problems. Figure 2.7 shows an assessment map that can guide you to blend information from a QPA and major nursing concerns.

Box 2.6   **Human Needs (Maslow)**

Clustering data according to *Human Needs (Maslow)* helps you set priorities.

- **Physiologic (survival) needs (Priority #1):** Food, fluids, oxygen, elimination, warmth, physical comfort.
- **Safety and security needs (Priority #2):** Things necessary for physical safety (e.g., a cane) and psychological security (e.g., a child's favorite toy).
- **Love and belonging needs (Priority #3):** Family and significant others.
- **Self-esteem needs (Priority #4):** Things that make people feel good about themselves and confident in their abilities (e.g., being well-groomed, having accomplishments recognized).
- **Self-actualization needs (Priority #5):** Need to grow, change, and accomplish goals.

Source: Summarized from Maslow, A. (2011). *Toward a psychology of being-reprint of the 1962 first edition.* Eastford, CT: Martino Publishing.

RULE   **Cluster data according to your purpose—how you cluster information influences what issues you identify.** To identify nursing issues, use a nursing model (e.g., Box 2.5). To identify signs and symptoms of possible medical problems, use a medical model (e.g., Box 2.7). To set urgent priorities, use the *ABC Approach* (Airway, Breathing, Cardiac, and Circulatory status). Remember that the ABC approach is NOT used when giving CPR (go to the American Heart Association at http://www.heart.org/HEARTORG/ for correct CPR procedures).

Box 2.7   **Clustering Data According to Body Systems**

The following helps you identify data that should be referred to the physician.

1. Cluster together a brief client profile (vital statistics), including the following: name, age, reason the individual is seeking health care, vital signs, any known medical problems or diagnoses, allergies, or problems with diet.
2. Cluster together any data you suspect may be abnormal for any of the following systems:
   - Respiratory system
   - Cardiovascular system
   - Nervous system
   - Integumentary system (skin)
   - Gastrointestinal system
   - Musculoskeletal system
   - Genitourinary system

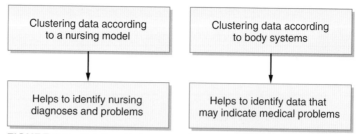

FIGURE 2.6   Relationship between clustering data and identifying health.

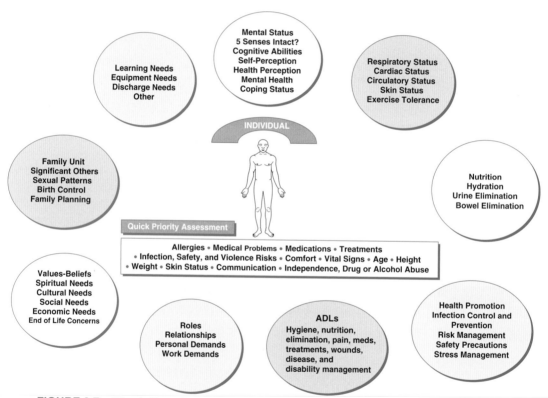

FIGURE 2.7   Alfaro-LeFevre Comprehensive Assessment Map. (© 2011 www.AlfaroTeachSmart.com)

CRITICAL THINKING AND CLINICAL REASONING EXERCISES

 Clustering Related Data

Example responses are provided at the end of the book (page 205).

1. Why is it important to organize data according to both a body systems framework and a nursing model?
2. Get a piece of paper and cluster the following data according to body systems (Box 2.7)

Patient Data
1. Age: 36
2. Married, has three small children
3. Occupation: Landscape architect and homemaker
4. Religion: Episcopalian
5. Medical diagnosis: Pneumonia
6. T: 100; P: 100; R: 28; BP: 104/68
7. States she is concerned about how her husband is caring for the children and that it is "tough on him."
8. States she feels weak and tired all the time but can't rest because she coughs all the time.
9. Appetite poor. Has eaten less than half of regular meals. Is forcing fluids well (1000 mL per shift).
10. States she smokes a pack of cigarettes a day.
11. States she has never been hospitalized (even gave birth at home).
12. States that all of the tests that have to be done make her nervous; she is worried about getting AIDS from needle sticks.
13. Lungs have bilateral rhonchi; she coughs up thick, yellow mucus.
14. Chest x-ray examinations show improvement over the past 2 days.
15. White blood cell count elevated at 16,000.

3. When you organized the previous data according to the categories of body systems or a nursing model, you may have found that some categories had no data listed. If this happens to you in the clinical area, what should you do?

Try This on Your Own

1. Draw a concept map of how the patient data in #2 above are related to one another. If you don't know how to draw a concept map, download "Nuts and Bolts of Concept Mapping" from http://www.alfaroteachsmart.com/handouts.html
2. **Understanding nursing models is central to gaining and understanding nursing approaches to patient care.** Compare and contrast the summaries of various nursing models (e.g., *Roy's Adaptation Model, Orem's Self-Care Model, Watson's Human Science and Care Model*, and others) posted at http://www.clayton.edu/health/nursing/nursingtheory

IDENTIFYING PATTERNS/TESTING FIRST IMPRESSIONS

After you cluster the data into related groups, you begin to get initial impressions of patterns of human functioning. But you must test these impressions and decide if the patterns really are as they appear. Testing first impressions involves:

● Deciding what's relevant
● Making tentative decisions about what the data suggest
● Focusing your assessment to gain more in-depth information to better understand the situations at hand.

Like the puzzle analogy, you put some of the puzzle pieces together and you think you know what the picture looks like. But sometimes those *last few pieces* surprise you with details that change the whole picture. Think about the following example in which a nurse clustered the following data together.

● **Objective data:** 72-year-old male; blind; bruises over right arm and on forehead
● **Subjective data:** "I use my cane to find my way, but I still bump into things."

The above suggests that there's a pattern of frequent injury related to blindness. However, there isn't enough information. You need to examine the data, decide what's relevant and irrelevant, and look for reasons why he has bruises. For example, think about the following relevant and irrelevant data in relation to this blind man's injuries.

● **Relevant:** elderly, blind, says he bumps into things, uses a cane, has bruises on right arm and forehead
● **Irrelevant:** male

The above supports the conclusion that the injuries are related to blindness. But you need to ask more questions, such as "Does he live alone, or is someone else responsible for his care?" and "Are the injuries really caused by blindness?" Perhaps he's falling down because of weakness or dizziness. After all, if he's using the cane correctly, do you think he'd bump himself all the time? These questions that come to mind when identifying patterns guide you to collect additional information to *test initial impressions* and describe the problems more clearly. For example, with the man just described, you could use probing questions to clarify how and why he keeps hurting himself. You may find that his injuries are related to fainting, poor cane use, abuse, or anticoagulant medications.

To focus your assessment on testing first impressions and gaining key data about patterns of health or illness, keep the following clinical reasoning principles in mind.

1. **Determine what's relevant and irrelevant:** Ask yourself what relevant information might be missing.
2. **Find out *why* or *how the pattern came to be*** (look for contributing factors). Remember that there's usually more than one contributing factor because health problems are complex.

REPORTING AND RECORDING

The final phase of *Assessment* is reporting and recording. This section focuses mainly on reporting and recording signs and symptoms during *an initial data base assessment*. Additional guidelines for reporting and recording during *Implementation* are addressed in Chapter 4.

Reporting and Recording Abnormal Findings

While policies and procedures for reporting and reporting information vary from place to place, this section gives general principles that apply to *all* communication and documentation.

Let's start by looking at the importance of reporting abnormal findings. Reporting anything you suspect might be abnormal does three things:

1. It promotes early diagnosis and treatment, even if you don't have the knowledge to diagnose the problems yourself.
2. It keeps others who are also accountable for your patient's care informed.
3. It helps you learn. You get help in determining whether the information is significant.

Recording abnormal data "flags" concerning symptoms and helps you and other caregivers to recognize downward trends in patient status.

Deciding What's Abnormal

There are many things to consider when deciding what's abnormal (e.g., age, disease process, culture, stress tolerance). If you're a novice, ask your preceptor, instructor, or direct supervisor to review your assessment data to be sure you're not missing something.

RULE **Before you can identify abnormal findings, you must know what's *normal* for each patient.** To decide if your patient has abnormal findings, compare your patient's data with accepted standards for normalcy. If the findings aren't *within normal limits,* consider them to be abnormal. For example, if you're caring for an adult and find a resting pulse of 110 beats per minute, this is *abnormal* because normal limits for an adult resting pulse is 60–100 beats per minute. Remember that normal limits may vary from one situation to another. For example, a pulse of 110 beats per minute may be normal for a child or for someone who's anxious, but abnormal for a sleeping adult who usually has a resting pulse of 60 beats per minute. Always ask yourself, "How normal is this for someone of this age, this culture, with this lifestyle, these problems, or in this situation?"

Box 2.8 shows questions to ask to determine normal versus abnormal.

Guidelines: Reporting and Recording

The following give basic principles and guidelines for making clinical decisions or answering test questions related to reporting and recording data.

- **Reporting and recording—accurate and complete communication and documentation—is an ongoing challenge for all nurses and health team members.** The most challenging times are during periods involving crisis, abnormal vital signs, and transfers. Yet, these are times when communication and documentation is extremely important.

Box 2.8	**Determining Normal and Abnormal**

Ask the Person
- Would you say this is normal or abnormal for you?
- What would you describe as normal for you?

Ask Yourself
- What's accepted as normal for someone who's this person's age? Physical stature? Culture? Developmental status?
- What's accepted as normal for someone who has:
  - This disease process?
  - This medication regimen?
  - This person's beliefs or cultural background?
  - This occupation, this socioeconomic level, this lifestyle?
- If I compare the data I've collected with the data gathered on admission (baseline data) or the data gathered in the past 24–48 hours, are there changes that reflect increasing problems?
- Are there too many slightly abnormal factors that, when put together, suggest an overall picture of abnormal?
- Is what the individual accepts as normal detrimental to his or her health?

- **Communication and documentation go hand in hand.** In many cases, nurses are required to complete specific documentation that they must use to guide verbal communication (e.g., SBAR Tool, Figure 2.5). Completing the documentation before giving verbal communications helps ensure that you have thought things through and have the most important information you need to report in front of you. The completed tool also serves as a reference to promote continuity of care after you leave.
- **Accurate and complete documentation is to crucial to** (1) communicating patient needs among caregivers, (2) giving safe effective care, (3) providing the data that help researchers improve care quality, and (4) creating a record that shows whether or not standards of care have been met.

RULE   **Always follow policies and procedures for (1) communicating patient status from one caregiver to another and (2) charting on the patient's record.** These policies and procedures are designed to ensure that the most significant patient information is reported and recorded in a timely way, keeping patients safe and guiding you to complete records that can help you avoid negligence suits.

- **When you suspect that patients need more qualified assessment or treatment than you're able to do, follow policies and procedures for activating the chain of command.** Be persistent—stay with the problems until your patients get the qualified help they need. Record all attempts to contact care providers about changes in patients' conditions. Include the names of anyone you notified, a brief summary of the reason for the call, and the care provider's response.
- **Use "Read Back" and "Repeat Back" rules in *all* important communications.** When you get verbal orders—or take down laboratory values—write down what you hear (or enter it into the computer), then *read it back* ("You want him started on amoxicillin 500 mg qid."). *Repeat back* key information ("You're not allergic to anything."). Ask others to repeat what you have said ("Can you repeat that so that I know we have it right?"). Passive strategies like *head-nodding* or *listening without saying anything* contribute to communication errors.
- **Complete documentation as soon as you can.** Charting when your memory is fresh promotes accuracy and helps you identify things you may have forgotten to do. Late charting leads to omissions and errors. In court, juries may interpret late charting to be substandard.
- **You may be required to record certain information within a specific time frame.** For instance, you may be required to record diagnoses present on admission—and that key interventions were initiated within specific time frames (e.g., patients with certain infections must be given an antibiotic within a certain time frame from admission).
- **Don't leave blanks on the patient record.** If a there's space to chart something, but it's not applicable to this particular situation, put "N/A" (stands for "not applicable").
- **Check organizational "do not use" lists** to be sure you don't use abbreviations that are potentially dangerous. You can find links to "do not use" lists at www. jointcommission.org.

- **Avoid terms that have a negative connotation** (e.g., "drunk," "disagreeable"). In court, they may convey a negative attitude on your part.
- **Keep it short, record the facts, and be specific.**

  EXAMPLE

  Wrong: Seems to have breathing problems and complains of chest pain.
  Right: Breath sounds diminished at lower left base. Complains of "piercing pain" with inspiration at the lower left base. Respirations 32, pulse 110, BP 130/90.

- **If you make an inference, support it with evidence.**

  EXAMPLE

  Wrong: Seems upset.
  Right: Seems upset. States that he's "not upset," but he doesn't make eye contact, uses only one-word answers, and states he doesn't "feel like talking."

- **If you get information from significant others,** list the name and the relationship of the person to the patient (e.g., "Wife states he's allergic to morphine.").
- **If you make a mistake, follow policies and procedures for correcting it.** *Never cover up the original words.* It may imply intent to cover up the facts, which is considered malpractice.
- **Guard the privacy of all records and communications—it's law.** Don't leave patient information open or displayed on the screen; log off the computer when you're not using it; retrieve printouts immediately.
- **Never share your password.** Change it often to avoid anyone guessing (most facilities automatically change it every 45–90 days). Tell your immediate supervisor if you suspect someone is using your code.
- **Find a way to *reflect* on your charting and the "big picture".** Whether you use a computer, smart phone, or other handheld device, don't just dump data in. Double-check for accuracy, look for trends, and *think* about what you record to identify patterns and ensure that your information is complete.

CRITICAL THINKING AND CLINICAL REASONING EXERCISES

 Reporting and Recording Significant Data

Example responses are provided at the end of the book (page 205).

1. **Practice identifying what's normal and abnormal.** Study the following data. In the space to the left, put "N" next to the normal data, "A" next to the abnormal data.

   a. States he usually has a bowel movement every other day.

   b. Temperature of 101°F.

    c. Pulse rate of 72 and regular (adult).

    d. Pulse rate of 150 (adult).

    e. Has hives over entire body.

    f. Infant cries as mother leaves the room.

    g. Patient complains of pain with urination.

    h. Grandmother suddenly does not recognize favorite grandchild.

    i. Grandmother says, "I can see okay as long as I wear my glasses."

    j. Infant cries, pulls at ears, and cannot be consoled by his mother.

2. **Learn how to ask relevant questions.** Having an assessment tool that's tailor-made to gain specific information in specific situations (e.g., in labor and delivery) is the key to getting relevant, complete data. Asking yourself *why each piece of information that the tool guides you to collect is required* helps you develop the clinical reasoning skill of *asking relevant questions*. Get an assessment tool from your instructor or preceptor (or use one of the ones in this chapter): Ask yourself why you have to record the data it requires entering.

Try This on Your Own

1. Decide where your documentation stands in relation to one of the following articles.
   Document It Right: Would Your Charting Stand Up to Scrutiny? by Maureen Habel, RN, MA http://ce.nurse.com/ce510/document-it-right-would-your-charting-stand-up-to-scrutiny/ Chizek, M. (2010). Documentation: Getting It Right. Accessed November 7, 2011, from http://nursing.advanceweb.com/Continuing-Education/CE-Articles/Documentation-Getting-It-Right.aspx
2. Discuss how you might use the comprehensive assessment map in Figure 2.7 as a worksheet to consider your patients most important concerns.
3. In a personal journal, with a peer, or in a group, discuss the implications of the following.

Voices

Documentation and Time Management: Help Wanted

I'm having trouble with electronic documentation. I like it, but I'm unsure how best use it. Mostly, I'm looking for time management advice. I find that if I record assessments in the patient rooms as I'm supposed to, I'm too distracted by the patient or someone else talking to me. In general, it seems to take too long. I begin my shift by checking on each patient and doing initial assessments. Then I pass meds, change dressings, and fulfill orders. I don't get to document until almost the end of the shift. I take notes during the shift and then enter what I did in the correct time slot. This is time-consuming, and if anything at all goes wrong, I'm still trying to catch up with documentation after my shift is over. I'm not getting to resolve care plan problems each shift, mainly because I forget to click on it. I'm struggling with this system. If anyone has developed a "system" that works well for electronic charting, time management, and reducing documentation errors, please share advice.

—Summarized from an online discussion on using electronic records.

Stepping into Peoples' Lives

As a nurse, you will step into people's lives... carry immense responsibility... see people at their worst, see people at their best... never be bored, always be frustrated... experience devastating failures, experience resounding triumphs... cry a lot, laugh a lot... see life begin and end... and KNOW WHAT IT IS TO BE HUMAN AND HUMANE[7]

—Melodie Chenevert, RN, BSN, MN, MA

Spiritual Needs Matter

Spirituality encompasses the whole of a person's being. Although many people do not subscribe to a recognized, organized system of beliefs—an established religion—virtually all humans are spiritual beings and uphold certain individual principles. These principles shape their view of themselves, the world, and God or a higher power.[8]

—Susan Richardson, RN, MS, CS

It Depends

I know my students are thinking critically when I ask them a question and they answer "It depends."[9]

—Toni C. Wortham, RN, BSN, MSN

Think About It

Nurse the Patients, Not the Computer

Patients call the rolling computer the nurse brings into their room "the nurse on a stick." Be sure that your patients know you're nursing *them*, not the computer.

Self-Efficacy Is Crucial to Learning New Skills

Believing in your ability to do what it takes to achieve your goals—called having self-efficacy—is extremely important when learning complex skills. If you have confidence problems, or see others with confidence problems, realize that this will cause brain-drain that will significantly affect your ability to learn. Deal with confidence problems early, by seeking or offering support. For more on self-efficacy, Google the term, and you'll find many resources.

This Chapter and NCLEX

- Stresses assessment and monitoring (safe, effective care):
  - Before, during, and after procedures.
  - Before, during, and after drug administration/
  - Setting priorities (what should you do first?)
- Initial = Assessment. When you see the word *initial*, the correct response is likely to refer to what needs to be *assessed*.
- If the question gives assessment data, decide whether you have *enough information* to make the diagnosis or to intervene. If you do not, the correct answer probably addresses what *else* needs to be assessed.
- When asked to prioritize, apply Maslow's Hierarchy of Needs (Box 2.6)
- Look for abnormal data in the question, as it influences decision making.

For complete test plan go to https://www.ncsbn. org/1287.htm

Key Points

- The safety, accuracy, and efficiency of all the other phases of nursing process depend on your ability to gather accurate, relevant, and complete assessment data.
- *Assessment* and *Diagnosis* are overlapping phases —you often move back and forth between these two phases.
- To promote sound clinical reasoning, your assessments should be purposeful, prioritized, focused, relevant, systematic, accurate, complete, and recorded in a standard way.
- Your ability to establish rapport, ask questions, listen, and observe is central to building a therapeutic relationship that's crucial to doing an assessment.
- Validating (verifying) data—ensuring that your information is factual and complete— helps you avoid making assumptions and jumping to conclusions.
- Figure 2.1 shows how the six phases of Assessment lead to *Diagnosis*.
- While ensuring complete data collection means gathering data *before you see the person, when you see the person*, and *after you see the person, always* consider *your direct patient assessment* to be your primary source of information.
- This chapter discusses three types of assessment—Data Base, Focus, and Quick Priority Assessments.
- Screening for risk factors that are known to create health problems is an important part of *Assessment*.
- Partnering with patients means moving from a paternalistic model ("we know what's best for you") to a partnership model ("we want you to be informed so that you can choose the best for you").
- The interview and physical assessment complement one another; you gain *subjective data* from what patients *state* and *objective data* from what you *observe* during your physical assessment.
- Physical assessment skills include inspection, auscultation, palpation, and percussion. Your physical assessment is incomplete until you check results of diagnostic studies.
- Standards mandate that you apply ethics principles and assess patients' cultural, spiritual, and communication needs.
- Your ability to identify cues and make correct inferences is influenced by your observational skills, your nursing knowledge, and your clinical expertise.

- To avoid missing nursing or medical problems, use both a body systems framework and nursing model to cluster data.
- Identifying patterns and testing first impressions help you avoid making assumptions and jumping to conclusions.
- Reporting and recording abnormal data in a timely way ensures early detection of patient problems and helps you learn how experts respond when patients have certain signs and symptoms.
- Scan this chapter for important rules, maps, and diagrams highlighted throughout; then compare where you stand in relation to the expected learning outcomes in the chapter opener (page 46).

References

1. American Nurses Association. (2010). *Nursing scope and standards of performance and standards of clinical practice* (2nd ed). Silver Springs, MD: nursesbooks.org.
2. U.S. Preventive Services Task Force. *Guide to clinical preventive services: Recommendations of the U.S. preventive Services task force*. Retrieved November 15, 2011, from http://www.ahrq.gov/clinic/pocketgd.htm
3. American Nurses Association. (2008). *Code of ethics for nurses with interpretive statements* (2nd ed). Silver Springs, MD: nursesbooks.org.
4. The Joint Commission. (2011). National patient safety goals. Retrieved November 15 from www.thejointcommission.com
5. The Joint Commission. (2011). Advancing effective communication, cultural competence, and patient- and. family-centered care: A roadmap for hospitals. Retrieved November 11, 2011, from http://www.jointcommission.org/Advancing_Effective_Communication/
6. Funk, M. (2011). As health care technology advances: Benefits and risks. *American Journal of Critical Care, 20*(4), 285–291.
7. Chenevert, M. (2010). *A student's road survival kit* (6th ed.). St. Louis, MO: Mosby-Elsevier.
8. Richardson, S. (2011). Making a spiritual assessment. Retrieved November 15, 2011, from http://ce.nurse.com/ce249-60/making-a-spiritual-assessment/
9. Wortham, T. (Verbal communication, May 8, 2011).

Chapter 3
Diagnosis

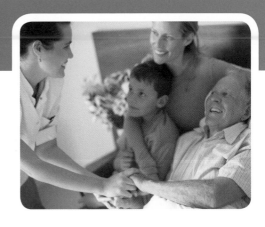

What's in This Chapter?

In this chapter, you learn principles of diagnostic reasoning—how to analyze the information you gathered during *Assessment* to correctly identify actual and potential problems. You learn *why diagnosis* is a critical point in the nursing process, how to make decisions about handling various nursing and medical issues, and how to avoid diagnostic errors. Stressing the importance of promoting independence and identifying human responses to diseases, treatments, and changes in life circumstances, you explore how nurses' responsibilities related to diagnosis are growing. You examine the impact of chronic diseases and disabilities on people's lives and learn the implications of moving from the *Diagnose and Treat* (DT) approach to the more proactive *Predict, Prevent, Manage, and Promote* (PPMP) approach. Finally, you examine how to (1) include patients as partners in the diagnostic process; (2) be a safe, effective diagnostician; and (3) map diagnoses to promote clinical reasoning.

ANA Standards Related to This Chapter

Standard 2   **Diagnosis.** The registered nurse analyzes the assessment data to determine the diagnoses or issues.[1]

Critical Thinking and Clinical Reasoning Exercises

Exercises 3.1   Diagnosis: Identifying Actual and Potential Problems; What ANA Standards Say; Diagnosis and Accountability; Increased Responsibilities Related to Diagnosis; Shifting to a Predictive Care Model; Nursing Versus Medical Diagnoses; Using Standard Terminology

Exercises 3.2   Becoming a Competent Diagnostician; Mapping Diagnoses/Problems; Identifying Potential Complications; Identifying Problems Requiring Multidisciplinary Care

Expected Learning Outcomes

After studying this chapter, you should be able to:

1. Apply basic principles of diagnostic reasoning—including taking specific steps to avoid diagnostic errors—to identifying actual and potential problems in the clinical setting.
2. Discuss the legal implications of the term *diagnosis*.
3. Explain why ANA standards state that nurses determine both *diagnoses* and *issues*.
4. Describe the relationship between *diagnosis* and *accountability*.
5. Explain the possible consequences of diagnostic errors.
6. Compare and contrast the *Diagnose and Treat* model with the *Predict, Prevent, Manage, and Promote* model.
7. Discuss how to use critical pathways and electronic decision support systems to identify actual and potential problems.

8. Make decisions about what standard terms to use in various clinical settings.
9. Identify resources that can assist you to make diagnoses.
10. Describe how to monitor to detect potential complications (PCs).
11. Make decisions about your responsibilities related to actual and potential nursing and medical problems.
12. Explain your role in relation to being a part of a multidisciplinary health team.
13. Draw diagrams or maps that give a clear picture of patient problems.
14. Give summary diagnostic statements using the PES and PRS methods.

DIAGNOSIS: IDENTIFYING ACTUAL AND POTENTIAL PROBLEMS

This chapter helps you learn the process of diagnostic reasoning—how to analyze the information you gained during assessment to identify actual and potential problems.

Continuing the puzzle analogy from Chapter 2, after completing *Assessment* you should have all the pieces of the puzzle (data). During *Diagnosis*, you decide what pieces go together to complete the puzzle and get a clear picture of your patient's problems, issues, and risks.

Remember from Chapter 2 that *Assessment* and *Diagnosis* overlap, as shown below.

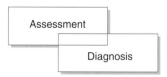

Diagnosis is a critical point in clinical reasoning for the following reasons.

1. **The purpose of *Diagnosis* is to clarify the exact nature of the problems and risks that must be addressed to achieve the overall expected outcomes of care.** If you don't completely understand the problems and what factors are contributing to them, how do you know what to do about them? If you don't pay attention to risks, how are you going to prevent problems?
2. **The conclusions you make during this phase affect the entire plan of care.** If your conclusions are correct, your plan is likely to be on target. If they aren't, your plan is likely to be flawed, maybe even dangerous.

RULE **Diagnosis—at least 50% of your challenge.** Determining actual and potential problems and clarifying their contributing factors requires in-depth critical thinking and is at least 50% of the challenge of developing the plan of care.

Figure 3.1 shows how *Assessment* leads to *Diagnosis*.

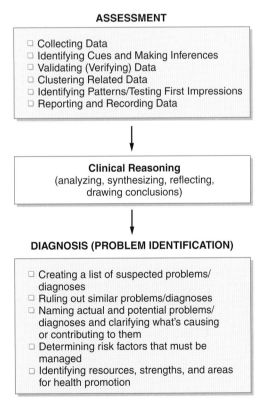

ASSESSMENT

- Collecting Data
- Identifying Cues and Making Inferences
- Validating (Verifying) Data
- Clustering Related Data
- Identifying Patterns/Testing First Impressions
- Reporting and Recording Data

Clinical Reasoning
(analyzing, synthesizing, reflecting, drawing conclusions)

DIAGNOSIS (PROBLEM IDENTIFICATION)

- Creating a list of suspected problems/ diagnoses
- Ruling out similar problems/diagnoses
- Naming actual and potential problems/ diagnoses and clarifying what's causing or contributing to them
- Determining risk factors that must be managed
- Identifying resources, strengths, and areas for health promotion

FIGURE 3.1 Key questions to determine whether you've identified a nursing diagnosis or multidisciplinary (collaborative) problem.

What ANA Standards Say

Because applying standards is central to clinical reasoning, let's look at what ANA standards say about *Diagnosis*: "The registered nurse analyzes the assessment data to determine the *diagnoses or issues*."[1] As a nurse, you'll deal with very specific problems (diagnoses) and ill-defined problems (issues).

Diagnosis and Accountability

A key starting point for learning about *Diagnosis* is understanding the concept of accountability—being responsible and answerable for something. Accountability may be moral, ethical, or legal—or all three of these. As a nurse, you have moral, ethical, and legal accountability for diagnosis, as indicated in the following rule.

RULE   **The term *diagnosis* implies that there's a situation requiring appropriate, qualified treatment.** This means if you diagnose an actual or potential problem, you must decide whether you're (1) qualified to make the diagnosis and (2) willing to accept responsibility for treating it. If you're not, you're accountable for getting qualified help. If you miss key problems or risks, you're *accountable* for what happens (e.g., if you don't recognize that your patient has risks for pressure ulcers and the area breaks down, you're accountable).

INCREASED RESPONSIBILITIES RELATED TO DIAGNOSIS

Laws and standards continue to change to reflect how nursing practice is growing. Depending on your qualifications and practice setting, you may have a wide range of responsibilities related to diagnosis and treatment of various health problems. The following are responsibilities related to diagnosis (problem identification) that are central to your role as a nurse.

- **Recognizing safety and infection-transmission risks and addressing these immediately** (e.g., if your patient is semiconscious, you make sure bed rails are up; if your patient has signs of a communicable disease, you begin isolation precautions according to policies and procedures).
- **Identifying human responses**—how problems, signs and symptoms, and treatment regimens *impact on patients' lives*—and promoting optimum function, independence, and quality of life (e.g., if your patient has debilitating arthritis, you identify the impact this problem has upon his daily life).
- **Anticipating possible complications** and taking steps to prevent them (e.g., if you identify that someone is at risk for aspiration, you must address the risks, e.g., turning the patient on his side).

- **Initiating urgent interventions**. You don't wait to make a final diagnosis if there are signs and symptoms indicating the need for immediate treatment (e.g., if your patient is hemorrhaging, notify the doctor immediately and start interventions aimed at correcting the problem—e.g., putting the patient flat in bed or applying pressure to the site that's bleeding).

RULE   Unless you're an Advanced Practice Nurse (APN), state laws prohibit you from making medical diagnoses. You are, however, accountable for giving high priority to assessing for—and reporting—signs and symptoms that may indicate the need for attention from a qualified professional. For instance, if your patient has signs and symptoms of a myocardial infarction (e.g., chest pain and shortness of breath), you're accountable for (1) suspecting that this could be the problem; (2) recognizing that it is a high priority; (3) doing what you can to address the problem (e.g., positioning the patient to facilitate breathing); and (4) reporting it immediately.

SHIFTING TO A PREDICTIVE CARE MODEL (PREDICT, PREVENT, MANAGE, PROMOTE)

As briefly addressed in Chapter 1, care delivery has shifted from "diagnose and treat (DT)," which implies we wait for signs and symptoms, to begin treatment to a predictive model—predict, prevent, manage, and promote (PPMP). The PPMP model is based on evidence. Thanks to research, we now know the typical course of most health problems. We also know how to *alter* the course through early intervention.

Using the PPMP model requires you to do three things[2]:

1. **In the presence of known problems,** predict the most common and most dangerous complications and take immediate action to (a) prevent them and (b) manage them in case they can't be prevented.

EXAMPLE

As a beginning nurse working in the emergency department, you admit a woman you suspect is having a heart attack. You report this problem immediately so that steps can be taken to control the problem and its PCs (e.g., an IV is inserted so that medications can be given to improve blood flow to the heart and prevent arrhythmias, if needed).

2. **Whether problems are present or not,** look for evidence of *risk factors* (things that evidence suggests contribute to health problems). If you identify risk factors, you aim to reduce or control them, thereby preventing the problems themselves.

EXAMPLE

You do an assessment and decide a teenage boy is in excellent health. However, you recognize that he has risky sexual behaviors. Recognizing that these behaviors put the young man at risk for contracting HIV and other sexually transmitted diseases, you focus on addressing the risky behaviors.

3. **In all situations,** ensure that safety and learning needs are met and promote optimum comfort, function, and independence.

EXAMPLE

You're caring for someone who is asthmatic and is being discharged after a colonoscopy. As you give discharge instructions, you assess the patient's learning needs related to care at home and initiate teaching as indicated. You also discuss how he manages his asthma. You may point out that a daily walking program strengthens muscles, prevents osteoporosis, improves endurance, is key to weight control, and promotes lung and cardiovascular function (all are especially important for asthmatics).

Using the PPMP model requires knowledge of not only health promotion but also disease process, treatment, and prognosis (the usual course and outcome of injury or disease). Keep in mind that the term *predict* in PPMP doesn't mean that a complication *will* happen. It's an assumption to think like this: *My patient has this problem, so I can predict that he'll have these complications.* The PPMP approach means you *anticipate* the possibility of complications and plan ways to monitor, detect, prevent, and manage them early.

Because many complications are medication related, remember the following rule.

RULE   Medication reconciliation—ensuring that you have a complete and up-to-date list of medications being taken—and monitoring patient responses to medication regimens are a major part of predicting and managing PCs.

Failure to Rescue and Rapid Response Teams

The issue of *failure to rescue* has brought new procedures that bring rapid response teams to the patient to ensure early intervention and adequate care. Failure to rescue is defined as a clinician's inability to save a hospitalized patient's life when he experiences a complication (a condition not present on admission).[3] For example, suppose nurses fail to monitor elderly patients closely for the common postoperative complications of respiratory, cardiac, and vascular problems (e.g., deep vein thrombosis). Then, suppose that as a result the patient experiences these complications. If the patient dies, this is considered *failure to rescue* because if nurses had detected signs and symptoms and responded appropriately (e.g., notified the doctor), these serious complications could have been avoided. The nurses were in a position of being able to rescue the patient from serious complications, but failed to do so. The work of researchers Clarke and Aiken at the University of Pennsylvania, as well as subsequent work by others, has significantly improved our ability to identify and correct issues related to monitoring for complications (called nursing surveillance).[4] Today we have *rapid response teams* that nurses can call to assist in assessing and managing patients who seem to be demonstrating concerning signs and symptoms. Rapid response teams, made up of specialists (e.g., doctors, respiratory therapist, pharmacists, and nurses), bring all the needed experts to rescue the patient to the bedside.

Many places have also initiated Code H (Code Help). Code H was developed when a child died when her family was unable to get her the attention they felt she needed (http://www.josieking.org/). If patients, families, and visitors are concerned that patient needs are not being met, they can call the operator to initiate a Code H. Examples of issues that may trigger a Code H include delays in getting pain medications, lack of communication, or worrisome signs and symptoms. Depending on the concern, appropriate professionals respond.

Provider-Preventable Conditions and Health Care–Acquired Conditions

Preventing complications is key to preventing pain and suffering and also essential to the financial survival of health care organizations. The Centers for Medicare and Medicaid Services (CMS) will not reimburse hospitals for provider-preventable conditions including health care–acquired conditions and other provider-preventable conditions. The following gives examples of provider-preventable conditions.[5]

- Foreign object retained after surgery
- Air embolism
- Blood incompatibility
- Stage III and IV pressure ulcers
- Falls and trauma, including fractures, dislocations, intracranial injuries, crushing injuries, burns, electric shock
- Catheter-associated urinary tract infection (UTI)
- Vascular catheter–associated infection
- Manifestations of poor glycemic control, including diabetic ketoacidosis, nonketotic hyperosmolar coma, hypoglycemic coma, secondary diabetes with ketoacidosis, secondary diabetes with hyperosmolarity
- Deep vein thrombosis (DVT) or pulmonary embolism (PE) following total knee replacement or hip replacement with pediatric and obstetric exceptions
- Surgical site infection following:
  - Coronary artery bypass graft (CABG)—mediastinitis
  - Bariatric surgery
  - Orthopedic procedures, including spine, neck, shoulder, elbow

Figure 3.2 summarizes key points of the predictive care model.

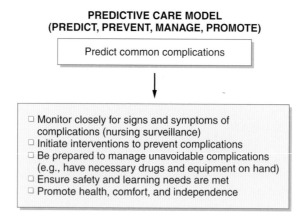

**PREDICTIVE CARE MODEL
(PREDICT, PREVENT, MANAGE, PROMOTE)**

Predict common complications

☐ Monitor closely for signs and symptoms of
   complications (nursing surveillance)
☐ Initiate interventions to prevent complications
☐ Be prepared to manage unavoidable complications
   (e.g., have necessary drugs and equipment on hand)
☐ Ensure safety and learning needs are met
☐ Promote health, comfort, and independence

FIGURE 3.2   Predictive care model. (© 2011 R. Alfaro-LeFevre Workshop Handouts.)

Clinical Pathways (Care Maps)

Clinical pathways—also called critical pathways or care maps, integrated care pathways, or care maps—are examples of using the PPMP model. These pathways are multidisciplinary, evidence-based standard plans that predict the day-by-day care required to achieve outcomes for specific problems within a certain time frame. (Appendix A shows an example critical pathway.)

There are advantages and disadvantages to using critical paths:

● **Advantages of Clinical Pathways**
1. Give outcome-focused, evidenced-based approaches.
2. Alert you to frequently encountered problems and predicted care for specific situations (e.g., repair of a fractured hip).
3. Help you learn the usual treatment course for common problems through repeated experience in using the paths with different patients.

● **Disadvantages of Clinical Pathways**
1. You may be so influenced by knowing major diagnoses and predicted care in advance that it's easy to become complacent, thinking, I already know the problems, so I don't have to worry too much about assessment.
2. Often patients have comorbidities, meaning they have other problems such as lung disease or significant mental health issues that aren't covered by the path.

When using critical pathways, keep an open mind and think independently. Always determine your patient's specific needs rather than assume she "fits" the typical critical path. Be sure that you consider all patient problems, not just those addressed on the path.

Point-of-Care Testing

To ensure early detection of problems, you'll be involved in point-of-care testing—diagnostic testing done by nurses at home or at the bedside. Examples of point-of-care tests are blood glucose measurement and testing stool for blood. In specialty units (e.g., intensive care), nurses may be accountable for complex point-of-care tests. Be sure you check with policies and procedures to know what tests you are responsible for doing and which ones are done by the laboratory. Be sure that you're prepared for point-of-care testing by practicing performing the tests if you're not doing them on a frequent basis (in many cases, you'll be required to pass competency tests to prove competence).

Disease and Disability Management

Today, more nurses are involved in disease and disability management, which involves helping patients with self-management of chronic problems at home (see Box 3.1). In disease and disability management, nurses are responsible for teaching patients how to manage their symptoms and helping them to navigate through the health care system. In partnerships with physicians, they provide the bulk of care by applying their knowledge and using evidence-based guidelines. Nurses are key players in reducing costs and improving quality of life by working with chronically ill patients to improve adherence to treatment plans, diets, and medications.

Informatics and Electronic Decision Support

Informatics—the use of computers to manage information and aid diagnosis and decision making—is a field that continues to evolve. As the use of electronic support tools grows, remember the rule on the next page.

Box 3.1   **Promoting Health in People With Chronic Health Problems***

Chronic diseases have a long course of illness. They rarely resolve spontaneously and they're generally not cured by medication or prevented by vaccine. Chronic diseases—such as heart disease, cancer, and diabetes—account for 7 of every 10 deaths and affect the quality of life of 90 million Americans. Chronic disabling conditions cause major limitations in activity for 1 out of every 10 Americans (25 million people). Prolonged courses of illness and disability often result in extended pain and suffering, as well as in decreased quality of life. Although chronic diseases are among the most common and costly health problems, they are also among the most preventable. Adopting healthy behaviors such as eating nutritious foods, being physically active, and avoiding tobacco use can prevent or control the devastating effects of these diseases. The United States can't reduce its enormous health care costs, much less its priority health problems, without addressing the prevention of chronic disease and disability in a more aggressive manner.

*Summarized from http://www.doh.state.fl.us/Family/chronicdisease/.

RULE   **While electronic support systems are valuable tools that can spot trends, facilitate problem identification, and help you learn, they're only as good as the human–computer interphase.** It takes experienced nurses who are knowledgeable in diagnostic principles and familiar with both the signs and symptoms of common patient problems and the technology to use electronic tools safely and effectively.

NURSING VERSUS MEDICAL DIAGNOSES

NANDA-I makes the following distinctions between nursing and medical diagnoses[6]:

- **"A nursing diagnosis is** a clinical judgment about actual or potential individual, family, or community experiences/responses to health problems/life processes. A nursing diagnosis provides the basis for selection of nursing interventions to achieve outcomes for which the nurse has accountability. Nursing diagnosis deals with human responses to bio-psycho-social stressors and/or health problems that a nurse is licensed and competent to treat." The main aim of studying what problems should be considered nursing diagnoses is to identify the independent nursing role—what nurses do beyond that of helping physicians treat patients. You can find frequently asked questions about nursing diagnosis at http://www.nanda.org
- **"Medical diagnosis** is a medical determination of disease or syndrome performed by a physician. The focus is on the disease process and the physical, genetic, or environmental cause of that process. Medical diagnosis deals with disease or medical condition or pathology (treating or curing)."

You may see the term "problem" is being used interchangeably with "diagnosis." This is because all diagnoses are health problems. Not all agencies use the term *nursing diagnoses*. Instead, they use the term *nursing problem*. Table 3.1 compares *nursing* and *medical diagnoses*. Figure 3.3 gives key questions to ask to determine if you identified a nursing diagnosis/problem or a medical or multidisciplinary problem.

USING STANDARD TERMINOLOGY

Using standard terms is required in all health care organizations. Using commonly understood terms is crucial to reducing errors and facilitating communication, documentation, and research. It's also crucial to developing electronic health records (EHRs). Because standard terminologies continue to evolve, this section helps you make decisions about what terms to use.

Table 3.1 Comparison of Nursing and Medical Diagnoses/Problems

Nursing Diagnoses/Problems	Medical Diagnoses/Problems
Main Focus	**Main Focus**
Human responses (the impact of disease, trauma, or life changes upon patients, families, and communities) Problems with functioning independently (activities of daily living) Quality of life issues (e.g., pain, ability to do desired activities)	Diseases, trauma, pathophysiology Complex behavioral and brain disorders Quality of life issues (e.g., pain, ability to do desired activities, but to a lesser extent than nursing—they often refer these types of problems to other disciplines)
Primary Manager of Problem	**Primary Manager of Problem**
Nurse (may use other resources such as physical therapy or physician expertise, but the nurse accepts primary responsibility for monitoring status and allocating resources)	Physician or advanced practice nurse (APN)
Definitive Diagnosis	**Definitive Diagnosis**
Authority to make the definitive diagnosis within the nursing domain	Authority to make the definitive diagnosis within the medical domain
Nursing Responsibilities	**Nursing Responsibilities**
Identification of signs, symptoms, and risk factors Early detection of actual and potential problems Initiation of a comprehensive plan to prevent, correct, or control the problems (nurse is the primary manager of the problems) Monitoring patient responses to nursing care	Identification of risk factors, anticipating potential complications (PCs) Monitoring to detect and report early signs or symptoms of PCs or change in status Initiating actions within the nursing domain to prevent or minimize the problems and their PCs Implementing medical orders (physician or APN is primary manager of the problems) and monitoring responses to treatment.

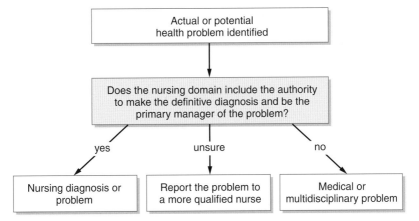

FIGURE 3.3 Key questions to ask to determine whether the problem you identified is a nursing diagnosis/problem or a medical or multidisciplinary (collaborative) problem.

ANA-Recognized Terminologies

The ANA recognizes 12 terminologies that support nursing practice. Table 3.2 gives examples of some of the groups who are on the ANA list of recognized terminologies. For complete list, go to http://www.nursingworld.org.

Developing nursing terminologies is important work. As terms are developed, the concepts are carefully studied, broadening nursing's knowledge base and proving

Table 3.2   Examples of Groups Developing Standard Terminologies

Group Name	Focus	Purpose
NANDA-I	Diagnoses	Increase the visibility of nursing's contribution to patient care by continuing to develop, refine, and classify phenomena of concern to nurses. **Web site**: http://www.nanda.org
Nursing Interventions Classification (NIC)	Interventions	Identify, label, validate, and classify actions nurses perform, including direct and indirect care interventions (interventions done directly with patients, e.g., teaching, and those done indirectly, e.g., obtaining laboratory studies). **Web site**: http://www.nursing.uiowa.edu
Nursing-Sensitive Outcomes Classification (NOC)	Outcomes	Identify, label, validate, and classify nursing-sensitive patient outcomes and indicators to evaluate the validity and usefulness of the classification and define and test measurement procedures for the outcomes and indicators. **Web site**: http://www.nursing.uiowa.edu
Home Health Care Classification (HHCC)	Diagnoses, Interventions, and Outcomes	Provide a structure for documenting and classifying home health and ambulatory care. Consists of two interrelated taxonomies: HHCC of Nursing Diagnoses and HHCC of Nursing Interventions. **Web site**: http://www.sabacare.com
International Classification for Nursing Practice (ICNP®)	Diagnoses, Interventions, and Outcomes	Capture nursing's contributions to health and provide a framework into which existing vocabularies and classifications can be cross-mapped, enabling comparison of nursing data from various countries throughout the world. **Web site**: http://www.icn.ch/icnp.htm
SNOMED CT (Systematized Nomenclature of Medicine—Clinical Terms)	Comprehensive clinical terminology	Integrate, link, and map terms from various disciplines such as medicine, nursing, and occupational therapy. **Web site**: http://www.nlm.nih.gov/research/umls/Snomed/snomed_main.html

Box 3.2	**Common Nursing Diagnoses/Problems in Adult Health***

- Risk for infection or infection transmission
- Risks to safety (e.g., falls)
- Risk for violence or self-harm
- Airway and breathing problems
- Impaired swallowing—risk for aspiration
- Altered mental status—confusion
- Impaired communication
- Pain-nausea-discomfort
- Anxiety–fear—coping issues
- Oral hygiene issues†
- Risk for pressure ulcer or impaired skin integrity
- Immobility—exercise Intolerance
- Altered nutrition
- Altered bowel elimination
- Altered urinary elimination
- Constipation
- Diarrhea
- Dehydration
- Patient education
- Self-care deficits (feeding, bathing, dressing, toileting)
- Altered sleep patterns
- Risks of allergic responses (e.g., latex, medications, environment)
- Smoking cessation
- Spiritual distress

*Partial list. Problems are summarized, rather than given specific labels.
†Linked to incidence of pneumonia.

nursing's worth by identifying exactly what problems nurses diagnose and manage, and what outcomes they can influence. Often, the nursing terminologies identify what it is that nurses do independently, beyond their role in implementing the medical plan of care.

Some nursing specialty organizations have identified the priority nursing problems that nurses in that particular setting diagnose, prevent, and manage. For example, the Association of Rehabilitation Nurses (ARN) addresses problems such as *self-care deficits, mobility issues, bladder issues, depression,* and *behavior management.*[7] The Association of periOperative Registered Nurses (AORN) addresses issues such as risk for *perioperative positioning injury, risk for electrical injury,* and *hypothermia.*[8] Box 3.2 gives examples of priority nursing diagnoses/problems in adult health nursing.

Standard Medical Terms

The medical discipline uses the *International Statistical Classification of Diseases and Related Health Problems* (commonly known as the ICD) published by the World Health Organization (http://www.who.int/classifications/icd/en/). Nurses also use these terms when addressing their patients' medical care.

How Do You Know What Terms to Use?

Depending on what setting you work in, you're likely to use terms from more than one of the accepted nursing, medical, and multidisciplinary terminologies. Whether or not a term is used is influenced by three things:

1. The clinical needs of each agency or setting
2. What terms have the best evidence to support their use (e.g., *dehydration* has been studied rigorously for years; *fluid volume deficit* has not)
3. What terms are best understood by patients and the multidisciplinary health care team (e.g., *patient education* is often used instead of *deficient knowledge*)

RULE **Know the required and forbidden terms at your agency or school.** As you move from setting to setting, take note of the terms used in standards, policies, protocols, and EHRs. Ask whether there is a list of recommended terms. These are the terms you must use. Also review the *Do Not Use List* (these are usually abbreviations that may not be understood by others). You can download the Institute for Safe Medical Practice's List of Error-Prone Abbreviations, Symbols, and Dose Designations from http://www.ismp.org (United States) and http://www.ismp-canada.org (Canada).

CRITICAL THINKING AND CLINICAL REASONING EXERCISES

Diagnosis: Identifying Actual and Potential Problems; What ANA Standards Say; Diagnosis and Accountability; Increased Responsibilities Related to Diagnosis; Shifting to a Predictive Care Model; Nursing Versus Medical Diagnoses; Using Standard Terminology

Example responses are provided at the end of the book (page 205).

1. How does diagnostic reasoning relate to clinical reasoning?
2. ANA standards state that nurses are accountable for treating diagnoses or issues. How do you know whether you're dealing with a diagnosis or an issue?
3. What is the relationship between diagnosis and accountability?
4. What is the relationship between managing risks and preventing and managing health problems?
5. When starting in a new clinical setting, how do you know what terms to use and what terms to avoid?
6. How do failure to rescue and nursing surveillance relate to the PPMP model?

Try This on Your Own

1. Take out a piece of paper and draw a line down the middle. On the left, list the advantages of using critical pathways. On the right, list the disadvantages. Then decide what you can do to overcome the disadvantages.
2. Discuss a time in your personal or professional life, when you misunderstood a problem or issue. How did you figure out that you misunderstood and what did you do about it?
3. Discuss the issues addressed in the following articles.
   - Friese, C., & Aiken, L. (2008). Failure to Rescue in the Surgical Oncology. *Oncol Nurs Forum, 35*(5):779–785. Accessed January 4, 2011, from *http://www.medscape.com/viewarticle/583103*
   - McGee, E. (2010). Failure to Rescue. Retrieved January 4, 2011, from *http://nursing.advanceweb.com/Article/Failure-to-Rescue.aspx*
4. Draw a map of how the following are related: diagnostic reasoning, nursing problems, medical problems, PPMP model, critical pathways, nursing surveillance, failure to rescue, accountability, diagnoses, issues, PCs.

BECOMING A COMPETENT DIAGNOSTICIAN

Becoming a competent diagnostician requires knowledge, experience, and an ability to dialogue about the diagnostic process with others. To be able to dialogue intelligently, you need a deep understanding of the following terms.

Key Terms Related to Diagnosis

Diagnose. To make a judgment and specifically name the actual and potential health problems or risk factors present, based on evidence from assessment.

EXAMPLE

After performing an assessment, the nurse diagnosed *Risk for Aspiration related to decreased level of consciousness and poor cough reflex.*

Diagnosis. In addition to referring to the second step of the nursing process, *diagnosis* means two things: (1) The *process* of diagnosing (e.g., "We learn diagnosis in the first semester") and (2) The *result* of the diagnostic process (e.g., "What's the diagnosis?").

Definitive Diagnosis. The most specific, most correct diagnosis.

> **EXAMPLE**
>
> If you're unsure whether your patient's urinary frequency is related to an infection, you refer the problem to a physician or APN so that a *definitive diagnosis* can be made. **Discussion:** Being *very specific* about the diagnosis is essential to being able to determine definitive treatment. Would you be satisfied with a diagnosis of "lung disease," or would you want a definitive diagnosis (e.g., pneumonia or asthma)?

Definitive Interventions. The *most specific* actions or treatments required to prevent, resolve, or manage a health problem.

> **EXAMPLE**
>
> If a patient has bacterial pneumonia, you encourage fluids, assist with coughing, and may administer oxygen. But, if you don't have the definitive intervention of giving an antibiotic that's effective against the specific bacteria causing the pneumonia, the problem will persist or even get worse.

Potential or Risk Problem. A health problem that may develop if preventive actions are not done.

> **EXAMPLE**
>
> *Risk for injury related to poor balance and history of frequent falls*. **Discussion:** Table 3.3 compares nursing responsibilities for actual, potential, and possible diagnoses/problems.

Competency. Having the knowledge and skills to identify problems and risks and perform actions safely and efficiently in various situations.

Table 3.3   Responsibilities for Actual, Potential, and Possible Nursing Diagnoses/Problems

Nursing Diagnoses/Problems	Nursing Responsibilities
Actual Diagnosis/Problem: The person's data show signs and symptoms or defining characteristics of the diagnosis. **Example**: Altered respiratory function *related to pain and thick mucus* as evidenced by coughing up thick mucus, statements of pain with deep inspiration, and shallow respirations.	Compare patient's signs and symptoms with the signs and symptoms of the diagnoses you suspect; determine the cause or related factors. Decide whether to treat independently or refer the problem.
Potential (Risk) Diagnosis/Problem: The person's data show the risk factors of the diagnosis/problem but **no** signs, symptoms, or defining characteristics. **Example**: *Potential altered respiratory function related to pain*	Control risk factors and monitor signs and symptoms of the problem.
Possible Diagnosis/Problem: You suspect a diagnosis/problem is present, but the person's data need more clarifying before you can decide whether the diagnosis/problem is present. **Example**: *Possible bowel elimination issues*	Collect more data to clarify whether or not the diagnosis/problem is present or whether there are related (risk) factors present.

EXAMPLE

After the first semester of nursing, the student demonstrated competency in giving medications. **Discussion:** You're considered competent to perform an action or diagnose health problems after you've completed appropriate courses and passed tests (clinical and theoretical) demonstrating competency.

Qualified. Being competent and having the authority to perform an action or give a professional opinion.

EXAMPLE

Suppose you know that you're competent to give IV drugs. If you start work in a new place, you have to check whether you have the authority to do so. **Discussion:** Authority to do assessments, perform nursing actions, and give professional advice comes under "scope of practice" and is derived from the following: laws (state practice acts), state boards of nursing, licensure, and certification; national and state standards; and facility standards, policies, procedures, and protocols. In Chapter 1, Figure 1.2 addresses how determining your scope of practice helps you determine your qualifications.

Nursing Domain. Activities and actions a nurse is legally qualified to do, either independently or under the direction of a medical doctor or APN. Also includes diagnoses that a nurse is qualified to make.

EXAMPLE

All nurses are accountable for diagnosing *risks for injury* independently. In critical care settings, nurses are accountable for diagnosing problems with heart rhythm and initiating treatment according to physicians' orders or protocols. **Discussion:** As you progress with your education and clinical experience, your nursing domain (practice scope) will include a wider range of responsibilities. You're accountable for maintaining competency within your practice domain.

Medical Domain. Actions a physician is legally qualified to do.

EXAMPLE

Performing surgery is in the medical domain so long as the physician is qualified to do so. **Discussion:** APNs now have more responsibilities for treating problems within the medical domain. When nurses take on responsibility for actions that previously belonged only to the medical domain, the actions must be approved by state rules and regulations. Boards of nursing usually issue position statements that describe what nurses can or can't do related to specific medical problems or procedures.

Outcome. The result of prescribed interventions. Usually refers to the *desired* result of interventions (that the problem is prevented, resolved, or managed); includes a specific time frame for when the outcome is expected to be achieved.

(EXAMPLE)

"By 3 days after total knee replacement surgery, the person will show no signs of infection, will be able to walk with a walker, and be ready to be discharged."

Signs. Objective (observable) data known to suggest a health problem (rashes and fever are signs).

Symptoms. Subjective (reported) data known to suggest a health problem (pain and fatigue are symptoms).

Cues. Signs and symptoms that prompt you to suspect the presence of a health problem (rashes, fever, pain, and fatigue) or a desire to improve health ("I want to improve my eating habits.").

Rule Out. To decide that a certain problem is *not* present.

(EXAMPLE)

You suspect that your patient has *activity intolerance related to sedentary lifestyle*. Before you can confirm this diagnosis, you must rule out whether your patient has cardiac or respiratory problems, which take priority.

RULE   **"Ruling out" is an important part of diagnostic reasoning.** Don't settle for the first problem you think of. Think of alternative problems that the data could represent. *Considering alternative problems and ideas* is a major critical thinking principle. In some cases, you may find that this is facilitated by electronic decision support: the computer will ask you to consider several other problems that your patient's data could represent.

Life Processes. Events or changes that occur during one's lifetime (growing up, becoming a parent, aging, losing a loved one, having surgery, dealing with illness or trauma, experiencing terminal illness). **Discussion:** Nurses are very involved in helping patients and families with transitions that occur across the lifespan.

Risk Factor or Etiology. Something known to cause, or contribute to, a problem (e.g., decreased vision is a risk factor for injury).

Syndrome. When a patient exhibits a cluster of signs and symptoms related to other major problems. For example, *posttraumatic stress syndrome*.

Fundamental Principles of Diagnostic Reasoning

To give you a sound foundation for diagnostic reasoning, this section gives fundamental principles for analyzing data and identifying actual and potential problems.

- **Always ask patients first.** Begin diagnosis by asking something like, "What are your main problems or goals today?" Creating partnerships with patients early in the diagnostic process ensures that you involve the most important member of the health care team (the patient).
- *Diagnosis* **involves comparing your patient's signs and symptoms with the "textbook picture" of the diagnoses or problems you suspect.** For example, if you suspect your patient has risk for pressure ulcer, compare your patient's risk factors with the risk factors listed under pressure ulcer in a reference. Keeping print or electronic resources that describe common diagnoses handy for quick reference will increase your accuracy and help you learn.
- **Become familiar with the priority problems often found in your particular practice setting (and what your responsibilities related to those problems are).** Box 3.2 lists common nursing diagnoses/problems in adult health. The inside back cover and facing page lists common PCs.

RULE   **While you will probably identify various priorities for your patient, remember to include the presence of any of the following on your list of priority problems:** (1) safety issues (e.g., risks for injury, violence, or harm), (2) potential for infection and infection transmission, and (3) patient education needs. Remember: "safety, infection, education."

- **Patients usually present with two or more related problems.** The first step is to identify the primary problem by looking at *relationships* among the problems. For example, someone may complain of both *anxiety* and *insomnia*. It's your job to determine the primary problem, which quite likely is *anxiety* (causing insomnia).
- **Problem identification is incomplete until you understand what's** *causing* **or** *contributing to* **the problems.** Keeping in mind the importance of focusing on the whole person, not just the disease(s), the following are steps to take to identify contributing factors.
  1. Ask patients and families questions like the following:
     - What do you think is causing this?
     - How do your symptoms impact on your ability to do daily activities?
     - How has your life changed?
     - How are you coping with these changes?
     - What resources (personal, community) might be able to help you?
  2. Determine whether there are factors related to developmental age, disease, treatment, or changes in lifestyle that may be contributing to the problem(s).
  3. Find out if there are cultural, socioeconomic, ethnic, environmental, or spiritual factors that may be contributing to the problem(s).
  4. Check your other resources for data collection (e.g., medical records, other health care professionals, literature review) to identify other factors that might be causing or contributing to the problem(s)?

RULE **Always ask yourself whether it's possible that the signs and symptoms you identify could represent a medical problem that needs in-depth assessment by a more qualified professional.** For example, if you're caring for someone with chronic constipation, be sure that this problem has been evaluated by a physician, as it's one of the signs of cancer.

- **Keep an open mind.** Avoid tendencies to be overly influenced by past experience or by information you gain from patient charts or others (e.g., you may assess someone whose chart reports a history of chronic arthritic back pain and fail to consider that an increase in back pain could signify something else, like a kidney problem).
- **When you suspect a certain problem, look for other signs, symptoms, and risk factors commonly seen with that problem.** For example, if you suspect infection because of localized pain and swelling, look for *other* signs of infection (fever, redness, heat, drainage).

RULE **"More than one cue, more likely it's true. More than one source, more likely of course."** This means the more signs and symptoms your patient has that mimic the signs of specific problem, the more likely it is that your patient has the problem.

- **If you miss a problem, mislabel a problem, or identify a problem that isn't there, you made a diagnostic error,** which may result in inappropriate, dangerous treatment. Box 3.3 summarizes the causes and risks of diagnostic errors. Box 3.4 addresses how to avoid diagnostic errors.
- **When you make a diagnosis, back it up with evidence.** Be ready to give the cues (signs, symptoms, risk factors) that led you to make the diagnosis. Rationale: Cues (signs, symptoms, risk factors) are like "key puzzle pieces"; if you don't have them, you can't complete the puzzle and label the problem. For example, your patient may have a productive cough and fever, causing you to suspect pneumonia. The doctor needs evidence from a chest x-ray examination, sputum culture, and white blood cell count to complete the puzzle and make the diagnosis.
- **Look for flaws in your thinking: (1) What other problems could the cues represent?** For example, if someone tells you he's been having increasing episodes of left shoulder pain due to an old injury, consider the possibility that this pain also could represent a cardiac problem. **(2) What could be influencing the status of the problems you suspect?** For example, you may have ruled out the possibility of infection because there is no fever, but when you check all the data, you realize that an antiinflammatory drug has been taken, reducing body temperature.
- **Although intuition is a valuable tool for problem identification, never make diagnoses on intuition alone:** look for evidence to verify your intuition. Diagnosis is based on evidence. Box 3.5 shows how to use intuition safely.

Box 3.3 | Causes and Risks of Diagnostic Errors

Causes of Diagnostic Errors

- Overvaluing the probability of one explanation or failing to consider all of the data because of a *narrow* focus. **Example**: Deciding that anxiety is related to psychological stress rather than considering whether there might be some physical problem, such as poor oxygenation, causing the anxiety.
- Continuing to *analyze* when you should be *acting* to get help (analysis paralysis). **Example**: Continuing to see if repositioning and emotional support help a breathing problem, even though they make no difference.
- Failing to recognize personal biases or assumptions. **Example**: Assuming that someone who doesn't bathe daily has a poor self-image.
- Making a diagnosis that's too general (not being specific enough in choosing a diagnostic label to name the problem). **Example**: Using *Impaired Urinary Elimination* instead of *Stress Incontinence related to weakness of bladder sphincter muscles*.
- Failing to include the correct diagnosis in the initial list of possible problems. **Example**: Listing the problems of *Noncompliance* but not including the possible problems of *Ineffective Coping or Ineffective Management of Therapeutic Regimen*.
- Rushing to get done, either when collecting or analyzing data. **Example**: Rushing through assessment or choosing any diagnosis that's close so you get to report on time, rather than communicating that you ran out of time to the next nurse.

Risks of Diagnostic Errors

When you miss a problem, mislabel a problem, or fail to fully understand a problem, you run the risk the following:

- Initiating interventions that actually aggravate the problems.
- Omitting interventions that are essential to solving the problems.
- Allowing problems to exist or progress without even detecting that they are there.
- Initiating interventions that are harmless but wasteful of everyone's time and energy.
- Influencing others that problems exist as described incorrectly.
- Harming patients and placing yourself in danger of legal liability

---

- **Diagnosis is incomplete until you identify not only the problems, but also strengths, resources, and areas for improving health** (Box 3.6 page 111).
- **Figure 3.4 (pages 112–113) shows the first two pages of a tool to guide diagnostic reasoning** (the complete tool can be downloaded from http://www. AlfaroTeachSmart.com). Using a tool like this consistently can help you develop good diagnostic reasoning habits. Figure 3.5 (pages 114–115) gives a patient self-assessment tool that can help patients think about their own signs and symptoms.

Box 3.4 — How to Avoid Diagnostic Errors

Do you:
- Take the time to be sure your data are accurate and complete?
- Compare your patients' signs and symptoms with the "textbook picture" of the diagnoses you suspect?
- Recognize your biases and avoid value judgments?
- Consider other problems that the cues might signify?
- Look for flaws in your thinking?
- Identify the cause(s) of the problem(s)?
- Include what the patient sees as problems?
- Choose the most specific diagnostic label(s) that best describes the problem(s)?
- Inform the patient (and significant others) of what you see as problems?
- Ask someone to double-check you when you're unsure?
- Validate the diagnosis with the patient?

Box 3.5 — How to Use Intuition Safely

1. Recognize that although you have no evidence that a problem exists, your intuition is sending up a red flag that says, "Something's wrong here," or "This patient needs help." Assess closely for existing signs and symptoms that validate the presence of the problem that you suspect. For example, say to the patient, physician, or another nurse, "My intuition tells me that …" or "I have the feeling that…"
2. If you know that something is wrong but can't put your finger on any specific problem, increase the frequency and intensity of nursing assessment to monitor closely for early detection of signs and symptoms.
3. Before you act on intuition alone, weigh the risks of the possibility of your actions causing harm (either aggravating the situation or creating new problems) against the risk of not acting at all (other than to monitor more closely).

Box 3.6	**Identifying Resources and Strengths**

1. **Ask the person and significant others questions like the following:**
   - Can you tell me some things about yourself that you view as strengths?
   - Can you think of any things that aren't really problems but you'd like to improve?
   - Who are your best resources; where do you get the best support?
2. **Cluster together data that indicate normal or positive functioning. Label these areas as strengths and share them with the person and significant others. For example, you might say, "You've made the decision to seek help, which is a healthy thing to do."**
3. **List the strengths that will help you to prevent or manage the identified problems.**

Examples
- **Physical strengths**: Exercises daily and has excellent cardiac and respiratory reserve; eats a balanced diet; demonstrates physical adaptation; upper torso and arms are powerful (compensating for paraplegia).
- **Psychological and personal strengths**: Is motivated; wants to be independent; relates understanding of care management and available resources; has good problem-solving skills.

MAPPING DIAGNOSES/PROBLEMS

Drawing a map of patient signs, symptoms, and problems helps you develop reasoning skills because you create a picture of relationships among patient data. Mapping has few rules, allowing you to focus on *thinking and relationships*, rather than rules. Your brain handles pictures better than words, especially if you're right-brain dominant.

Figure 3.6 (page 117) shows a structured mapping worksheet, which guides you to consider key information when making diagnoses. This worksheet asks you to consider *all possible factors* contributing to the problem. When you consider *all factors contributing* to a problem, you can then scan the worksheet and decide who is in charge of managing what contributing factors. For example, if your surgical patient is taking steroids, you need to remember that this puts him at risk for poor wound healing. You then know to be more diligent about monitoring the wound. You can also discuss with the physician what, if anything, can be done about the steroid regimen.

Figure 3.7 (page 118) shows a fill-in-the-blank diagnosis summary map. Figure 3.8 (page 118) shows the completed diagnosis summary map. If you need more information on mapping, download *Nuts and Bolts of Concept Mapping* from http://www.alfaroteachsmart.com/handouts.html

(continues on page 116)

COMPREHENSIVE ANALYSIS TOOL
A Guide For Diagnostic Reasoning

NOTE: This tool is designed for *beginning students* caring for *adult patients.* It's NOT intended to replace standard assessment tools. Rather, it helps you to do in depth analysis to *draw conclusions* about the data recorded on them. While this guide prompts you to approach diagnosis systematically, it doesn't replace the need for independent judgment or ability to apply basic principles of diagnostic reasoning. Using this tool consistently will help you develop habits that prioritize your approach to diagnosis.

Keeping a nursing focus – to maximize patient self-mangement, bio-psychosocial function, and quality of life – this tool guides you through the process of thinking about nursing concerns. It incorporates principles from *Gordon's Functional Health Patterns and Maslow's Human Needs*, and considers *Healthy People 2010* recommendations (for example, screening for depression). It also prompts you to check for disease often included in disease management programs. To help you prioritize, it lists questions according to things you need to think about early (for example, whether signs and symptoms are caused by a communicable disease).

This tool patient self-assessment tools are available for download free *for personal or student use only* at: www.AlfaroTeachSmart.com (click on *Publications*, then *Handouts*).

1. List admitting diagnoses and current major problems according to patient, family, and medical records.

2. Rule out presence of infection or communicable disease (check for fever, fatigue, pain, redness, heat, swelling, drainage, exposure to communicable disease or toxic substance; travel to foreign country).

3. Rule out whether patient signs and symptoms are actually medication problems. Consider all drugs taken (including over-the-counter and herbal remedies). Use **SODA** to jog your mind:

   ☐ **S**ide effects?

   ☐ **O**ver dosage?

   ☐ **D**rug interactions?

   ☐ **A**llergy or **A**dverse reactions?

4. Rule out whether the patient's signs and symptoms are actually allergic responses or due to history of surgery or trauma. Check for patient history of the following:

☐ Arthritis or Back Pain	☐ Depression/mental	☐ Thyroid Disease
☐ Asthma or other Lung Disease	health problems	☐ Vascular/Circulation
☐ Bleeding problems	☐ Diabetes	Problems
☐ Cancer (Breast, Prostate, Other)	☐ Hypertension	☐ Wound Healing Problems
☐ Congestive Heart Failure/	☐ Infection/HIV	☐ Surgery/trauma
Heart Disease	☐ Obesity	☐ Skin problems
☐ Neurological problems	☐ Kidney Disease	☐ Other diseases/problems:

5. Has there been significant weight loss or gain? (Consider as far back as 6 weeks. Remember that unexplained weight loss may indicate serious medical problems like cancer, or diabetes; unexplained weight gain may indicate serious kidney, heart, or thyroid disease).

A

FIGURE 3.4   First two pages of a tool to guide diagnostic reasoning. Download full tool from http://www.AlfaroTeachSmart.com. (© 2011 AlfaroTeachSmart.com.)

**COMPREHENSIVE ANALYSIS TOOL
A Guide For Diagnostic Reasoning**

6. Determine smoking pattern and possible role in current problems:

Yes   ☐ Quit Smoking   ☐ Never Smoked   Packs per day _____

7. For pre-menopausal women (age <55 years), rule out possibility of pregnancy (many drugs, diagnostic studies, or treatments affect the fetus).

8. Rule out whether there are problems (or risk factors for problems) with any of the following.

(Circle those that apply)

☐ Breathing or coughing, or oxygenation?	Yes	No	AR[1]	Pos[2]
☐ Blood pressure, pulse, bleeding, circulation?	Yes	No	AR	Pos
☐ Pain, stiffness or discomfort?	Yes	No	AR	Pos
☐ Body temperature or sweating?	Yes	No	AR	Pos
☐ Ability to think or perceive environment?	Yes	No	AR	Pos
☐ Communication (seeing, hearing, or speaking)?	Yes	No	AR	Pos
☐ Eating, digestion, or nutrition?	Yes	No	AR	Pos
☐ Bowel elimination?	Yes	No	AR	Pos
☐ Dehydration, edema or electrolyte imbalance?	Yes	No	AR	Pos
☐ Movement, range of motion, or activity intolerance?	Yes	No	AR	Pos
☐ Rashes, skin problems, ulcers, or tissue perfusion?	Yes	No	AR	Pos
☐ Sleeping?	Yes	No	AR	Pos
☐ Infection (vulnerable or contagious to others)?	Yes	No	AR	Pos
☐ Safety (risk for injury or falls; weakness or seizures)?	Yes	No	AR	Pos
☐ Anxiety, coping or managing stress?	Yes	No	AR	Pos
☐ Drug or alcohol dependence?	Yes	No	AR	Pos
☐ Growth and developmental challenges?	Yes	No	AR	Pos
☐ Life style changes (e.g., divorce, moving, new parent)?	Yes	No	AR	Pos
☐ Roles, relationships, sexuality, or self-esteem?	Yes	No	AR	Pos
☐ Patient or family education needs?	Yes	No	AR	Pos
☐ Difficulties at home or work?	Yes	No	AR	Pos
☐ Ability to do desired, as well as necessary activities?	Yes	No	AR	Pos
☐ Personal, religious, spiritual, cultural beliefs?	Yes	No	AR	Pos
☐ Ethical issues?	Yes	No	AR	Pos
☐ Socio-economic issues?	Yes	No	AR	Pos

HOW TO PRIORITIZE: **Problems usually present in a cluster** (patients rarely have only one problem). Before going on to the next page, study the above and consider *relationships* among the problems. For example, if pain is contributing to depression or movement problems, **pain** is a major problem. If you're unsure whether a problem is present, ***collect more data.***

AR[1] = At Risk for problem (no signs and symptoms present, but risk factors are evident).

Pos[2] = Possible problem (insufficient data, but you suspect a problem).

B

FIGURE 3.4   (*Continued*)

COMPREHENSIVE PATIENT SELF-ASSESSMENT TOOL

Note to Our Patient Partners: Because YOU are the one who knows yourself best, we want you to be informed, involved participants in your care. Studies show that people who are actively involved in making decisions about their care are likely to have the best results. In all aspects of your care, remember the following Speak Up steps, from the Joint Commission:

- ☐ Speak up if you have questions or concerns. If you don't understand, ask again. It's your body and you have a right to know.*
- ☐ Pay attention to the care you are receiving. Make sure you're getting the right treatments and medications by the right health care professionals. Don't assume anything.
- ☐ Educate yourself about your diagnosis, your testing procedures, and your treatment plan.
- ☐ Ask a trusted family member or friend to be your advocate.
- ☐ Know what medications you take and why you take them. Medication errors are the most common health care errors.
- ☐ Use hospitals, clinics, surgery centers, or other types of health care organizations that have undergone rigorous on-site evaluations against established state-of-the-art quality and safety standards, such as that provided by the Joint Commission.
- ☐ Participate in all decisions about your treatment. You are the center of the health care team.

1. Get focused and help us prioritize. Tell us your 3 biggest problems or concerns.

2. Please list any current medical problems.

3. List any surgery you have had, including date when surgery was done.

4. (For women) when was your last menstrual period?

5. Do you smoke? ☐ Yes ☐ Quit Smoking ☐ Never Smoked   Packs per day _____

If you smoke, we strongly recommend that you stop. Please ask for our information on smoking cessation. You CAN do it, with help!

*Speak Up approach is courtesy of the Joint Commission, http://www.jointcommission.org/

FIGURE 3.5   First two pages of a patient self-assessment tool. Download full tool from http://www.AlfaroTeachSmart.com. (© 2011 AlfaroTeachSmart.com.)

COMPREHENSIVE PATIENT SELF-ASSESSMENT TOOL

6. Do you drink alcohol?   □ Yes   □ No   If yes, how much per week?

7. List allergies and medications (include over-the-counter and herbal drugs).

Allergies:

Drug	Dose	Taken how often?	Last dose?	Prescribing doctor?

8. Could any of your symptoms be medication related? Remember SODA:

□ Side effects?

□ Over dosage?

□ Drug interactions?

□ Allergy or Adverse reactions?

9. What screening tests have you had done (e.g., colonoscopy, mammography)?

10. Put an X on the box, if you have a family history of any of the following:

□ Cancer   □ Glaucoma

□ Heart disease   □ Mental health problems

□ Diabetes   □ Other

□ Hypertension

11. Children/Pregnancies:

Number of living children you have: ____ Number deceased: ____

For women, number of pregnancies you have had: ____

FIGURE 3.5   (*Continued*)

H.M.O. (HELP ME OUT)®

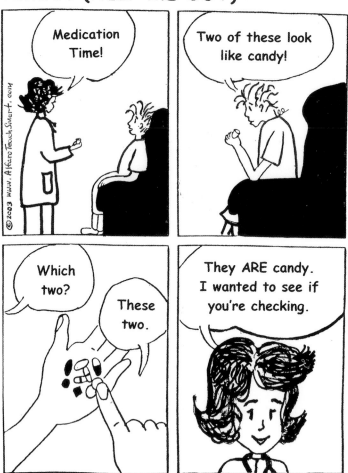

BE ON YOUR PATIENTS' S.I.D.E.*

Use S.I.D.E. to remember overarching care principles.

S-   **Safety and comfort.** Make safety and comfort top priority.

I-   **Infection prevention.** Be alert to infection risks; wash your hands; teach patients to do the same.

D-   **Dignity.** Help patients maintain self-respect; ensure privacy.

E-   **Engage and educate.** Involve patients and families in making decisions; teach them what they need to know to be independent.

*© 2012 www.AlfaroTeachSmart.com

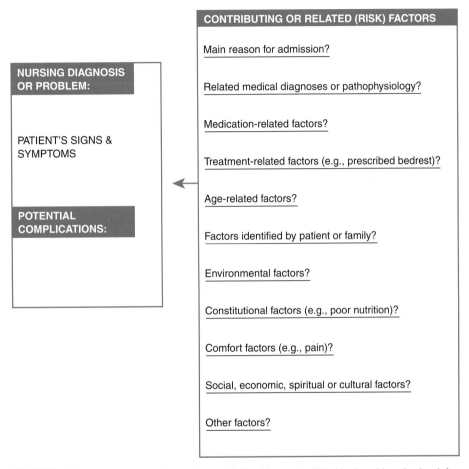

DIAGNOSIS/PROBLEM MAPPING WORKSHEET

INSTRUCTIONS: To get a clear picture of the diagnoses you identify, use this page to map your problem and all related or contributing factors.

NURSING DIAGNOSIS OR PROBLEM:

PATIENT'S SIGNS & SYMPTOMS

POTENTIAL COMPLICATIONS:

CONTRIBUTING OR RELATED (RISK) FACTORS

Main reason for admission?

Related medical diagnoses or pathophysiology?

Medication-related factors?

Treatment-related factors (e.g., prescribed bedrest)?

Age-related factors?

Factors identified by patient or family?

Environmental factors?

Constitutional factors (e.g., poor nutrition)?

Comfort factors (e.g., pain)?

Social, economic, spiritual or cultural factors?

Other factors?

FIGURE 3.6 Structured mapping worksheet that guides you to fill in blanks addressing key information you should consider when making diagnoses.

Recording Summary Statements Using the PES or PRS Format

You may be required to record diagnostic statements that summarize the most important elements of the diagnoses you identify. In this case, the PES (Problem, Etiology, Signs and Symptoms) format—also called the PRS (Problem, Related Factors, and Signs and Symptoms) format—is often used.

To record an *actual* diagnosis—when you identified signs and symptoms of the diagnosis—use the PES or PRS format to create a three-part statement as follows:

1. State the problem.
2. Use "related to" to link the problem and its etiology—the cause or related (risk) factors.
3. Give the signs and symptoms that show evidence that the diagnosis is present, using the words "as evidenced by."

FILL-IN-THE-BLANK DIAGNOSIS SUMMARY MAP

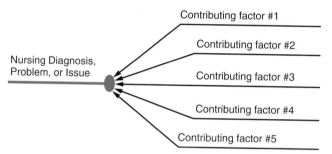

FIGURE 3.7   Fill-in-the-blank diagnostic summary map.

COMPLETED DIAGNOSIS SUMMARY MAP

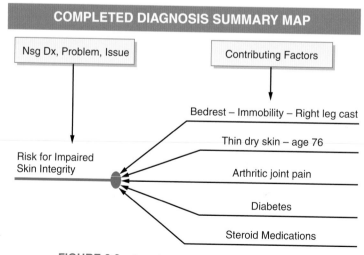

FIGURE 3.8   Completed diagnostic summary map.

Box 3.7   Diagnosis/Problem Summary Statement

Summary statements help communicate most important pieces of the diagnosis in a concise way.

_____ related to _____ as evidenced by _____.

> **EXAMPLE**
>
> Impaired communication related to language barrier as evidenced by speaking and understanding only German.

To record potential or risk diagnosis—when you've identified risk factors, but no actual signs and symptoms of the diagnosis—use a two-part statement that describes the problem and risk factors present.

> **EXAMPLE**
>
> *Risk for pressure ulcer* related to immobility and excessive sweating

When writing summary statements, be as explicit as you can. Add "secondary to" after the PES (or PRS) format to address key related problems.

> **EXAMPLE**
>
> Right heel *pressure ulcer* related to immobility and loss of sensation *secondary to* spinal cord injury.

Box 3.7 shows a fill-in-the-blank diagnosis summary statement.

IDENTIFYING POTENTIAL COMPLICATIONS

Identifying PCs is a complex skill for beginning nurses to develop. The following guidelines help you be a safe clinician when learning how to identify PCs.

Guidelines: Identifying PCs

- **Until you feel confident identifying PCs, report all abnormal data.** What may seem like an isolated cue to you may prompt a more experienced person to be concerned.
- **List present and past health issue.** Past health problems often point to undiscovered current health problems. For example, if your patient has a history of depression or violence, consider whether these problems could be present now.
- **Look for medication-related complications.** Review all medications taken and be sure the medication regimen is up-to-date. Use the following memory-jog (SODA).

Use SODA to Consider Medication-Related Complications

- S—Side effects?
- O—Overdose/toxicity?
- D—Drug interactions?
- A—Allergy or Adverse reaction?
- **Consider the possibility of allergic responses** (to dyes used in diagnostic studies, or other environmental factors).

RULE **Tell your patients to be sure their caregivers know about their allergies—stress that first time allergic response may be mild, but subsequent exposure could be significantly worse.** Follow policies for recording allergies in ways that flag this problem for all caregivers. You'll probably need to put a special wrist band on the patient as well as record allergies in a specific place in the patient record.

- **Be aware of recent diagnostic or treatment modalities—** determine whether there are commonly associated PCs (e.g., thrombi, emboli, and bleeding are PCs of cardiac catheterization).

RULE **To identify potential complications, ask, What could go wrong? What problems might occur and what do the signs and symptoms of these problems look like?** For instance, if you have someone with fractured ribs, look up fractured ribs in a resource and find out what the common complications are (in this case, *pneumothorax* and *hemothorax*). Then look up the signs and symptoms of *pneumothorax* and *hemothorax* (chest pain, increased respirations, feelings of not getting enough air, decreased breath sounds)?these are signs and symptoms you need to be monitoring your patient for.

- **Remember that the onset of complications is often subtle.** Signs and symptoms gradually worsen over a period of time. Always compare your data with data charted by others over the past 24–48 hours (sometimes longer). For example, if you get a temperature reading of 99.6°F, compare the reading with temperatures over the past 24–48 hours.
- **Review critical paths, policies, procedures, protocols, and standards that address your patient's situations** (e.g., management of chest tubes). These often guide you to assess for specific signs and symptoms you must report to monitor for PCs.
- **Read patient records** (e.g., nursing assessments, medical history and physical assessment, progress notes, consultations, diagnostic studies). Be sure you're aware of past medical problems as they often point to future ones.
- **In complex situations, check with the primary care physician or APN.** For example, say something like, "Are there any specific signs and symptoms you want us to report?"

IDENTIFYING PROBLEMS REQUIRING MULTIDISCIPLINARY CARE

Let's finish this chapter by addressing problems that require multidisciplinary care. Multidisciplinary care—a team approach that brings medical, nursing, and allied health care professionals together to work with patients and families to give expert, patient-centered is the norm today. With this care model, treatment plans are developed collaboratively and care delivery is a shared responsibility.

Being part of a multidisciplinary team means being keenly aware that you don't work in isolation. When you have complex patient situations, ask, Is it likely that this patient will be able to reach the desired outcomes in the expected time frame using only nursing expertise for care management? If the answer is "no," initiate appropriate referrals. For example, if the outcome for a healthy woman having a hysterectomy is "will ambulate the first day after surgery," you could expect to achieve this outcome using nursing resources alone. However, if the woman has other coexisting problems, for instance, difficulty walking due to neuromuscular problems, consider requesting a physical therapist's involvement with planning and managing ambulation.

CRITICAL THINKING AND CLINICAL REASONING EXERCISES

Becoming a Competent Diagnostician; Mapping Diagnoses/Problems; Identifying Potential Complications; Identifying Problems Requiring Multidisciplinary Care

Example responses are provided at the end of the book (page 206).

1. Choosing from the following words, fill in the blanks in the following statements.

qualified	knowledge	accountability	practice
referring	domain	experience	dialogue

   a. Becoming a competent diagnostician requires _____, _____, and being able to _____ intelligently with others about the process.

   b. The term diagnoses implies that there's a problem that requires _____ treatment.

   c. You are qualified to diagnose a specific health problem independently so long as they are within your _____ of _____ and you're willing to accept _____ for managing both the problem and contributing factors. If not, you are accountable for _____ the suspected problem to a qualified professional.

2. Check your knowledge of key terms. Choosing from the following, write the term(s) that best match the definitions listed below (write the term next to the letter).

diagnose   diagnosis   medical domain   definitive diagnosis
potential problem   accountable   competency   being qualified
life processes   nursing domain   outcome   medical diagnosis
nursing diagnosis   definitive interventions   risk factor
signs   symptoms   rule out   human response
multidisciplinary problem

_____ **a.** Something known to contribute to (or be associated with) a specific problem

_____ **b.** A health problem for which someone is at risk

_____ **c.** The judgment that's made after drawing conclusions about assessment data; also may refer to the skill of analyzing data to make a judgment

_____ **d.** To make a judgment and identity and name risk factors, problems, or strengths based on evidence from an assessment

_____ **e.** Being responsible and answerable for something

_____ **f.** Range of activities and actions that a physician is legally qualified to initiate or prescribe

_____ **g.** Range of activities and actions that a nurse is legally qualified to initiate or prescribe

_____ **h.** Usually refers to the desired or expected result of interventions (i.e., the problem is prevented, resolved, or controlled)

_____ **i.** How individuals respond to health problems or life processes, an important concern for nurses

_____ **j.** Events or changes that occur during one's lifetime (e.g., becoming a parent, aging, separations, losses)

_____ **k.** The most specific diagnosis

_____ **l.** The most specific actions required to prevent, resolve, or control a problem

_____ **m.** A problem requiring definitive diagnosis and treatment by a qualified physician; APNs also may treat some of these problems

_____ **n.** Having the knowledge and skill to perform an action or give opinions

_____ **o.** Having the competency and authority to perform an activity

_____ **p.** Objective (observed) data known to be associated with a diagnosis

_____ **q.** To decide that a problem isn't present

_____ **r.** Subjective (reported) data associated with a diagnosis

_____ **s.** A clinical judgment about an individual, family, or community

_____ **t.** A complex patient situation that requires collaborative management by nursing, medicine, and other health care professionals

3. Check your understanding of the difference between nursing and medical problems: Write "N" in front of the phrases that describe characteristics of nursing problems.

_____ a. Deals mostly with problems with anatomy and physiology.

_____ b. Includes health problems related to independence and activities of daily life.

_____ c. Definitive diagnosis is often validated by medical diagnostic studies.

_____ d. Deals with actual or potential problems with human responses to disease or life changes.

_____ e. Signs and symptoms don't improve after nurse-prescribed interventions are performed.

_____ f. Signs and symptoms improve after nurse-prescribed interventions are performed.

4. Apply the PPMP model. Imagine that you admit a 58-year-old man who hit his head in a fall at home. A concussion was ruled out, but he has a bad leg laceration which was sutured in the emergency department. Vital signs are normal. He is allergic to penicillin.

   a. What key piece of information is missing?

   b. What complications may occur?

   c. What will you monitor to detect if those complications are beginning to happen?

5. Write a diagnostic summary statement for the following problem by filling in the blanks that follow:

   Problem: Mrs. Cappelli has a temperature of 101° F. She sleeps a lot and has had only a glass of juice to drink today. She states that her appetite is poor, that she feels weak, and that she hasn't voided since last night. She is on a regular diet and has no fluid restrictions. _____ related to _____ and _____ as evidenced by _____ and _____.

Try This on Your Own

With a partner or in a group:

1. Determine the implications of the following statement: *Diagnosis* involves comparing your patient's signs and symptoms with the "textbook picture" of the diagnoses or problems you suspect.

2. A good way to start learning how to identify nursing problems is to "work backward": start with a list of common problems and assess every one of

your patients for those problems (soon the problems and their related signs, symptoms, and risk factors will become familiar to you). Assess your patients for the presence of all the problems listed in Box 3.2.

3. Discuss your responsibilities related to medical, nursing, and multidisciplinary problems (use Table 3.1 and Box 3.2 as a guide).

4. Discuss the following article in relation to the importance of identifying risks.
   - Midgley, M., Aumiller, L., & Moskowitz, M. (2011). Every Nurse is a Risk Manager retrieved November 27, 2011, from http://ce.nurse.com/ce105-60/every-nurse-is-a-risk-manager/

5. In a personal journal, with a peer, or in a group, discuss the implications of the following *Voices* and *Think About It* entries.

Voices

Diagnosis—Like Working a Human Puzzle

Taking care of a really sick patient is like working a human puzzle. The complex technology, machines, tubes, drains, medications, blood products, multisystem problems, and difficult surgeries make patient care pretty intimidating... but also challenging and exciting. I remember a case that perplexed the medical staff. A patient suddenly went downhill several days after open-heart surgery. Doctors and nurses searched for postsurgical complications, but found no answers. Having seen it in a patient once before, I raised the possibility of an *ischemic bowel*. They examined the abdomen, did a bowel resection, and saved his life. The doctor wrote to thank me, (Summarized from Rains, L. (2010).Thinking like a nurse. Retrieved November 28, 2011, from http://www.ajc.com/jobs/thinking-like-a-nurse-640609.html.)

All Problems Aren't Created Equal—Determine the Cause

To treat health problems, be sure that you understand the underlying causes. For example, studies support that chronic wounds are biologically different from acute wounds like surgical incisions, so they require different treatment. Acute wounds usually follow the body's "healing cascade" in a predictable and orderly way. However, chronic wounds such as pressure ulcers are usually "stalled" in the inflammatory healing phase, requiring an intensive evidence-based treatment plan. Local wound care without the correct supportive care, based on etiology or cause, won't work![9]

—*Elizabeth A. Ayello, PhD, RN, CS, CWOCN*

Predicting, Preventing, and Managing Violence

The most significant factor that helps to predict, prevent, and manage violence is asking about history of previous violent episodes. With angry or high-risk patients, ask questions like, "Have you ever felt out of control or been violent in the past?" ... "What do you do when you feel like you're losing control?" ... "What can we do when you're feeling like this?"[10]

—*Nico Oud, RN, MNSc, Dipl. N. Adm*

Safety Climate Prevents Patient and Nurse Injuries

Researchers led by Jennifer Taylor, PhD, MPH, found that a unit's safety climate was associated with both patient and nurse injuries, suggesting that patient and nurse safety may be linked outcomes. For each 10-point increase in a unit's average safety climate score, the odds of decubitus ulcer declined by 44%–48% and the odds of nurse injury declined by 40%–45%.[11]

 ## Think About It

No Patient Is a Critical Path

Critical paths are developed for specific problems, not specific people.

Confirmation Bias: A Common Diagnostic Mistake

Be aware of confirmation bias (the human tendency to see only evidence that supports your initial beliefs). For example, a colleague who is an APN works in an emergency department. A staff nurse reported that she had just admitted a patient with appendicitis and reported all the signs and symptoms that supported the diagnosis of appendicitis (e.g., right-sided abdominal pain, vomiting, and a family history of appendicitis). When the APN examined the patient, she asked about last menstrual period, did an exam, ordered studies, and found a life-threatening ectopic pregnancy.

The Difference between Expert and Novice Diagnosticians

The main difference between expert clinicians and students is that experts have a wealth of experience "in their heads." They readily probe deeply to rule in or out problems. On the other hand, students have confidence issues—major "brain-drains"—and they're overwhelmed by an inability to narrow down information to what's most important. Experts who think out loud, explaining how they made their diagnoses, are invaluable to helping students gain diagnostic reasoning skills.

This Chapter and NCLEX

- When prioritizing diagnoses, physiologic needs rise above all others. Airway issues and abnormal lab values are top priority. Risks for suicide, safety, and infection are a priority too.
- Be sure to note and connect all the data in the question. Missing a key piece of information may point you to the wrong answer. *Analysis* and *application* are the highest-level questions.

- Expect questions on all major nursing specialties, as well as advance directives; infection, injury, and error prevention; family systems, cultural diversity, legal rights, and responsibilities; bioterrorism, disaster response, human sexuality, and mental health.

Key Points

- This chapter focuses on diagnostic reasoning—how to analyze the information you gained during assessment to identify actual and potential problems.

- The term *diagnosis* has legal implications. It implies that there's a problem that requires qualified treatment.

- When you identify a problem, you must decide whether you accept accountability for treating it. If you don't, then you must report the problem to the appropriate qualified professional.

- Including patients as partners in diagnosis is a key to preventing errors and identifying the priority problems.

- Depending on your qualifications and practice setting, you may have a wide range of responsibilities related to diagnosis, prevention, and treatment of various health problems.

- Care delivery has shifted from a DT model to a predictive model—PPMP model. With PPMP, you anticipate potential complications and intervene early.

- Nursing surveillance, a key part of the PPMP model, is essential to preventing failure to rescue incidents.

- Point-of-care testing and disease and disability management is becoming an important nursing role.

- When using critical pathways, always determine patients' specific needs rather than assume that they "fit" the typical critical path. Be sure that you consider all patient problems, not just those addressed by the path.

- Depending on what setting you work in, you're likely to use terms from more than one of the accepted nursing, medical, and multidisciplinary terminologies. Whether or not a term is used is influenced by three things: (1) the clinical needs of each agency or setting, (2) what terms have the best evidence to support

their use, (3) and what terms are best understood by patients and the multidisciplinary health care team.

- Patients usually present with two or more related problems. The first step is to identify the primary problem by looking at *relationships* among the problems.

- Problem identification is incomplete until you understand what's *causing* or *contributing to* the problems.

- To be a competent diagnostician—and know how to respond to NCLEX questions and electronic decision support programs—make the principles and rules of diagnosis, as addressed in this chapter, habits of thinking.

- Developing your diagnostic reasoning skills requires knowledge, experience, and knowing how to dialogue about the process. For this reason, you need a deep understanding of key terms related to diagnosis, as addressed in this chapter.

- Mapping diagnoses and considering all factors that contribute to the diagnoses is the key to identifying a comprehensive treatment plan.

- If you're required to write a summary statement to describe the diagnoses you make, use the PES (problem, etiology, signs and symptoms) or PRS (problem, risk or related factors, signs and symptoms) method.

- With multidisciplinary care, treatment plans are developed collaboratively with various health care professionals, and care delivery is a shared responsibility. You're responsible for reporting problems that are likely to require more than nursing expertise to resolve, thereby initiating a multidisciplinary approach.

- Scan this chapter for important rules, maps, and diagrams highlighted throughout, then compare where you stand in relation to the expected learning outcomes in the chapter opener (page 90).

References

1. American Nurses Association. (2010). *Nursing: scope and standards of practice* (2nd ed.). Silver Spring, MD: Nursesbooks.org.
2. Alfaro-LeFevre, R. (2013). *Critical thinking, clinical reasoning, and clinical judgment: A practical approach* (5th ed.). Philadelphia, PA: Saunders-Elsevier.
3. McGee, E. (2010). Failure to Rescue. Advance for Nurses. Retrieved November 25, 2011, from http://nursing.advanceweb.com/Article/Failure-to-Rescue.aspx
4. Friese, C., & Aiken, L. (2008). Failure to Rescue in the Surgical Oncology. *Oncol Nurs Forum*, 35(5):779–785. Retrieved November 25, 2011, from http://www.medscape.com/viewarticle/583103
5. Centers for Medicare and Medicaid Services. (2011). Provider preventable conditions. Retrieved November 25, 2011, from http://www.medicaid.gov
6. NANDA-I (Web site). Retrieved November 26, 2011, from http://www.nanda.org
7. Association of Rehabilitation Nurses. (2007). *Evidence-based rehabilitation nursing: Common challenges and interventions.* Glenview, IL: Author.
8. Association of periOperative Registered Nurses. (2010). *The perioperative nursing data set* (3rd ed.). Denver, CO: Author.
9. Ayello, E. Personal communication, 2010.
10. Oud, N. Personal communication, 2010.
11. Taylor, J., Dominick, F., Agnew, J., et al. (2011). Do nurse and patient injuries share common antecedents? An analysis of associations with safety climate and working condition Web Site of BMJ Quality and Safety. Accessed November 25, from http://bit.ly/scZ7lb

Chapter 4
Planning

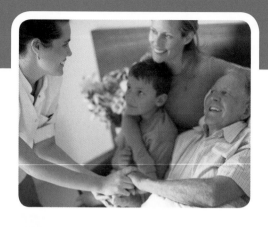

What's in This Chapter?

Having a recorded plan that's focused, specific, and up-to-date makes the difference between safe, effective care and care that's haphazard (even dangerous). This chapter examines clinical reasoning during the development of a comprehensive plan of care (Chapter 5 addresses the ongoing planning needed during *Implementation*). Here, you gain the skills you need to be able to record a plan that meets practice standards and promotes safe, efficient patient care. You learn the four main purposes of the plan of care and how to determine what problems *must* be recorded. You gain an understanding of key principles and rules of developing patient-centered outcomes and individualized nursing interventions. Finally you clarify your responsibilities related to recording a comprehensive plan, including how to use standard and electronic plans.

ANA Standards Related to This Chapter[1]

Standard 3	**Outcome Identification.** The registered nurse identifies expected outcomes for a plan individualized to the health care consumer or the situation.
Standard 4	**Planning.** The registered nurse develops a plan that prescribes strategies and alternatives to attain expected outcomes.
Standard 5a	**The registered nurse coordinates care delivery.**
Standard 5b	**Health Teaching and Health Promotion:** The registered nurse employs strategies to promote health and a safe environment.

Critical Thinking and Clinical Reasoning Exercises

Exercises 4.1	Setting Priorities; Clarifying Expected Outcomes Developing; Outcome Statements; Recognizing Affective, Cognitive, and Psychomotor Outcomes
Exercises 4.2	Determining Interventions; Individualizing Interventions Based on Problems and Outcomes; Monitoring to Detect Potential Complications; Ensuring the Plan Is Adequately Recorded

Expected Learning Outcomes

After studying this chapter, you should be able to:

1. Describe four main purposes of the plan of care.
2. Explain how the memory-jog EASE helps you remember the four main care plan components.
3. Explain the difference between initial and ongoing *Planning*.
4. Name five things that influence setting priorities.
5. Decide how to set priorities when doing a comprehensive plan of care.
6. Give four reasons why specific, measurable outcomes are the key to effective planning.
7. Address the relationship of outcomes to accountability.
8. Make decisions about accepting accountability.
9. Explain the importance of considering clinical, functional, and quality-of-life outcomes.
10. Discuss how to use standard plans (e.g., critical paths and electronic plans).
11. Explain the role of case management in planning efficient, cost-effective care.
12. Discuss how to weigh risks and benefits when determining nursing interventions.
13. Determine specific interventions that are tailored to each particular patient situation.
14. Develop and record a comprehensive plan of care that's individualized to the patient.
15. Evaluate patient records to determine if the plan of care is adequately documented.

CLINICAL REASONING DURING PLANNING

Focusing on *initial comprehensive planning*, this chapter addresses the thinking you need to do when developing and recording a plan of care. Chapter 5 addresses the ongoing, day-to-day planning you do during *Implementation*, including how to make decisions about delegating care.

Here, you learn how to ensure that the plan you record promotes safety and efficiency, meets practice standards, and clearly communicates care management to all those involved in your patient's care. Remember from Chapter 1 that *Planning* is a key part of *Implementation* (putting the plan into action).

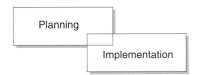

Having a well thought-out plan is the key to safe and effective *Implementation*.

FOUR MAIN PURPOSES OF THE PLAN OF CARE

The recorded plan of care serves four main purposes:

1. Directs care and documentation
2. Promotes communication among caregivers, thereby facilitating continuity of care.
3. Creates a record that can later be used for evaluation, research, and legal reasons.
4. Provides documentation of health care needs for Medicare, Medicaid, and other insurance reimbursement purposes

To meet the above purposes, the plan of care must have the following components.

Major Care Plan Components

The word **EASE** helps you remember the four main care plan components.

E-Expected outcomes
A-Actual and potential problems
S-Specific interventions
E-Evaluation/progress notes

Figure 4.1 shows the phases of *Planning* in context of developing an initial plan of care.

PLANNING

☐ Attending to Urgent Priorities
☐ Clarifying Expected Outcomes (Results)
☐ Deciding Which Problems Must Be Recorded
☐ Determining Individualized Nursing Interventions
☐ Making Sure the Plan Is Adequately Recorded

FIGURE 4.1   *Planning* in context of developing a comprehensive plan of care.

RULE   Because the plan of care guides interventions performed during *Implementation*, you are responsible for making sure that the plan is:

1. Individualized to the patient, considering each patient's unique circumstances (e.g., their age, health state, culture, values, capabilities, desires, and resources); and
2. Recorded according to facility policies and procedures.

STANDARD AND ELECTRONIC PLANS

In many cases today, you'll have standard and computer plans to guide your care. These tools are helpful because they spot trends and jog your mind to think about key things you need to include in the plan. For example, if you enter the diagnosis of diabetes, the computer asks you to consider whether you need to send a consultation to the dietary department to have someone come and discuss nutritional needs with the patient. However, remember the following rule.

RULE **Standard and electronic plans are guides that generally—but not always completely—apply to individual patient situations.** You are responsible for discriminating about what does and doesn't apply and for individualizing care accordingly.

PATIENT SAFETY, INFECTION PREVENTION, AND PAIN AND RESTRAINT MANAGEMENT

As we continue to focus on evidence-based care, national standards for important issues such as patient safety, infection prevention, and pain and restraint management are constantly refined and updated. These standards give focused, comprehensive approaches to preventing unnecessary patient suffering. They also help reduce costs. When you go to a new clinical setting, ask for policies and procedures related to things like pain management; use of restraints; and prevention of infection, falls, and errors. Be sure you incorporate these standards into the plan of care.

ATTENDING TO URGENT PRIORITIES

Some nurses will tell you *Planning* starts with setting priorities. Others will tell you it starts with clarifying outcomes. In a way, they're both right. To start, you do two things:

1. Determine urgent problems (e.g., those requiring immediate attention) before taking the time to clarify outcomes.
2. After you handle urgent priorities, determine overall expected results—usually called discharge outcomes—so you know how to prioritize in context of the big picture of patient care.

For example, think about how your priorities might differ if you were planning care for patients with the two following discharge outcomes.

● Three days after surgery, the patient will be discharged home, able to demonstrate wound care.
● Three days after surgery, the patient will be discharged to a skilled nursing facility for wound care and medical management.

If your patient will manage his own wound care at home, you give teaching about wound care a high priority. But if your patient is being discharged to a skilled nursing facility, teaching about wound care is a lower priority—it may even be inappropriate, depending on patient capabilities.

You can see that identifying desired outcomes early in the planning phase is crucial to setting priorities. To help you know how to identify urgent priorities, Box 4.1 gives basic principles for setting priorities.

| Box 4.1 | **Setting Priorities: Basic Principles** |

1. **Choose a method of assigning priorities and use it consistently.** For example, for identifying initial urgent priorities, some nurses use the ABC method (make sure the patient has no threats to his Airway, Breathing, or Circulation).
2. **Maslow's Hierarchy of Needs is helpful for setting priorities, especially when answering question on the NCLEX exam.**
   - **Priority 1. Physiologic needs**—Life-threatening problems (or risk factors) posing a threat to physiologic needs (e.g., problems with breathing, circulation, nutrition, hydration, elimination, temperature regulation, physical comfort)
   - **Priority 2. Safety and security**—Problems (or risk factors) posing a threat to safety and security (e.g., environmental hazards, fear)
   - **Priority 3. Love and belonging**—Problems (or risk factors) posing a threat to feeling loved and a part of something (e.g., isolation or loss of a loved one)
   - **Priority 4. Self-esteem**—Problems (or risk factors) posing a threat to self-esteem (e.g., inability to perform normal activities)
   - **Priority 5. Personal goals**—Problems (or risk factors) posing a threat to the ability to achieve personal goals
3. **Problems usually present in a cluster**—Study the relationships among the problems to determine major priorities. Assign high priority to problems that contribute to other problems. For example, if someone has chest pain and difficulty breathing, pain management is a high priority because pain causes increased stress and oxygen demand.
4. **Use the following strategies for setting priorities:**
   - **Ask, "What problems need immediate attention and what could happen if I wait until later to attend to them?"** Take immediate appropriate action to initiate treatment as indicated (e.g., notify the charge nurse and initiate actions to reduce the problem).
   - **Identify problems with simple solutions and initiate actions to solve them (e.g., correcting someone's position to improve breathing, calling a friend or family member to come in).** Sometimes, simple actions have a big impact on physiologic and psychological status.
   - **Develop an initial problem list, identifying actual and potential problems, and their causes, if known.** This method gives you a visual record you can reflect on to check whether you're missing anything and also to think about whether one problem might be contributing to another.

CLARIFYING EXPECTED OUTCOMES (RESULTS)

ANA standards stress the importance of identifying outcomes early in the nursing process.[1] In fact, remember that *outcome identification* is so important that it's sometimes considered to be a "sixth step" in the nursing process. As with NCLEX, in this book, we address it as an integral part of *Planning*.

Expected (desired) outcomes are descriptions of what the patient will be able to do when the plan is terminated. Outcome descriptions serve three main purposes:

1. **Outcomes are the "measuring sticks" for the plan of care.** You determine the success of the plan by finding out if the patient achieved the expected outcomes. For example, suppose you have the expected outcome of "the patient will be discharged able to change his own dressing by the 3rd day after surgery." On the 3rd day after surgery, is he able to do this?
2. **Outcomes direct interventions.** For example, in the above case, you need to make sure that the patient gets the teaching and practice needed to do dressing changes.
3. **Outcomes are motivating factors.** Having a deadline for getting things done gets everyone working toward the same deadline.

> **RULE**   **Early clarification of expected outcomes (the benefits expected to be seen in each particular patient after interventions are done) is the key to safety and efficiency.** If you don't know the expected outcome of interventions—and the evidence that supports that you're likely to achieve those outcomes—then you shouldn't be intervening at all, because you haven't thought it through.

Goals, Objectives, Outcomes, and Indicators

The terms goals, objectives, outcomes, and indicators are sometimes used interchangeably—but they are slightly different. *Goals and objectives* refer to *intent* (e.g., "Our goal or objective is to teach this person about diabetes."). *Outcomes and indicators* refer to specific *results* (e.g., "How will we know if this person actually learned what he needs to know about diabetes?"). The following example shows an example outcome with corresponding indicators.

EXAMPLE

Example Outcome	Corresponding Indicators
Maintains intact skin	Skin shows no signs of discoloration or irritation
	Control of risk factors recorded on chart per protocol (e.g., patient has adequate nutrition and hydration, repositioned hourly, skin care every 8 hours)

Principles of Patient-Centered Outcomes

To pass NCLEX and succeed in the clinical setting, be sure that you're familiar with the following principles of patient-centered outcomes.

1. **Outcomes describe the specific benefits you expect to see in the patient after care has been given.** In some cases, for example, with a newborn, outcomes may describe what you expect to see in a caregiver (e.g., "Father will safely bathe the newborn.").
   - Short-term outcomes describe early expected benefits of nursing interventions (e.g., "Will be able to walk to the bathroom unassisted by tomorrow.").
   - Long-term outcomes describe the benefits expected to be seen at a certain point in time after the plan has been implemented (e.g., "Will be able to walk independently to the end of the hall three times a day within 10 days after surgery.").
2. **Outcomes may relate to problems or interventions.**
   - Outcomes for problems state what you expect to observe in the patient when the problems are resolved or controlled (e.g., "The patient will have no signs or symptoms of infection.").
   - Outcomes for interventions state the benefit you expect to observe in the patient after an intervention is performed (e.g., if you suction someone's tracheostomy, you expect that breath sounds will be clearer after suctioning). If you can't clearly identify the benefits you expect to see in the patient after nursing care, then you shouldn't be intervening.
3. **To determine outcomes for problems, state the problem,** then reverse the problem to describe the improvement in the problem you expect to see (Figure 4.2).

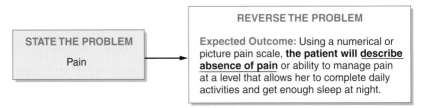

FIGURE 4.2   How to determine outcomes for problems.

4. **To determine outcomes for interventions,** state the specific benefits you expect to observe in the patient after the intervention is performed (Figure 4.3).
5. **To create very specific outcomes,** include the following components.

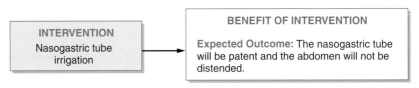

FIGURE 4.3   How to determine outcomes for interventions.

Five Components of Outcome Statements

Subject: Who is the person expected to achieve the outcome (e.g., patient or parent)?

Verb: What actions must the person take to achieve the outcome?

Condition: Under what circumstances is the person to perform the actions?

Performance criteria: How well is the person to perform the actions?

Target time: By when is the person expected to be able to perform the actions?

(EXAMPLE)

"Parents will bathe newborn in room independently by 5/8."

6. **Use measurable verbs** (verbs that describe things you can see, feel, smell, or hear). For instance, suppose you write an outcome for a woman that says, "Will understand how to use sterile technique." The word *understand* is vague and therefore not measurable. Ask yourself, How can we really know if she understands? The only way you can really know how well she understands is if she actually verbalizes or demonstrates sterile technique. The following are examples.

(EXAMPLES)

Measurable verbs: identify; list; walk; describe; hold; cough; state; exercise; verbalize; perform; will lose; will gain; demonstrate; express; communicate; has an absence of

Non-measurable verbs: know; understand; learn; feel; think; appreciate

7. **Consider** affective, cognitive, and psychomotor outcomes, as described in the following bullets.
   - **Affective domain:** Outcomes associated with changes in attitudes, feelings, or values (e.g., deciding eating habits need to be changed).
   - **Cognitive domain:** Outcomes dealing with acquired knowledge or intellectual skills (e.g., learning the signs and symptoms of diabetic shock).
   - **Psychomotor domain:** Outcomes dealing with developing motor skills (e.g., mastering how to walk with crutches).

(EXAMPLES)

Verbs used in cognitive, psychomotor, and affective outcomes:

- **Affective Domain:** Express, share, communicate, relate, explain
- **Cognitive Domain:** Discuss, describe, list, identify, explain, demonstrate
- **Psychomotor Domain:** Perform, walk, administer, demonstrate

The following guidelines help you clarify expected outcomes.

Guidelines: Determining Patient-Centered Outcomes

1. Start by asking patients first (e.g., "Tell me two to three major goals you'd like to achieve.").
2. Be realistic and consider:
   - Patient's health state, overall prognosis
   - Expected length of stay
   - Growth and development
   - Patient values and culture
   - Other planned therapies for the patient
   - Available human, material, and financial resources
   - Risks, benefits, and current scientific evidence
   - Changes in status that indicate you need to modify usual expected outcomes
3. Carefully compare your patient's actual situation with the standard plans and decide whether the outcomes are appropriate to your patient's particular situation.
4. In complex cases, develop both short- and long-term outcomes. Use short-term outcomes as stepping stones to the long-term outcomes.
5. Be sure the outcomes and indicators are measurable: that they describe something you can hear, see, feel, or smell in the person to demonstrate that the outcomes are achieved.
6. Box 4.2 shows how to use SMART to remember five main characteristics of well-developed goals and outcomes.

Relationship of Outcomes to Accountability

Determining outcomes helps you decide accountability for resolving problems. Study Figure 4.4, which helps you decide your accountability after you identify expected outcomes.

Box 4.2	**Memory-jog SMART for Goals and Outcomes**

SMART helps you remember characteristics of well-developed goals and outcomes.
S–Specific
M–Measurable
A–Agreed upon by all parties
R–Realistic
T–Time bound

Source: P. SMART: Characteristics of Good Objectives. Retrieved January 16, 2012, from *http://www.scn. org/cmp/modules/pd-smar.htm*

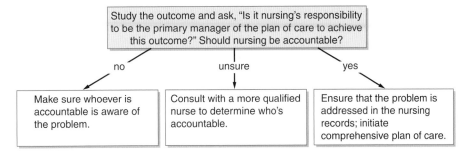

FIGURE 4.4   Determining outcomes helps you decide accountability for resolving problems.

Clinical, Functional, and Quality-of-Life Outcomes

Considering clinical, functional, and quality-of-life outcomes helps ensure that you develop a comprehensive plan that addresses the most important desired results.

Clinical outcomes describe the expected status of health issues at certain points in time, after treatment is complete. They address whether the problems are resolved or to what degree they are improved.

EXAMPLE CLINICAL OUTCOMES

- Chest tube out 3rd postoperative day
- Lungs clear, absence of signs of infection 2 days after admission
- Able to demonstrate wound care 3 days after surgery

Functional outcomes describe the person's ability to function in relation to the desired usual activities.

EXAMPLE FUNCTIONAL OUTCOMES

- Four days after total knee replacement, Mr. Palmer will be discharged to a rehabilitation facility able to perform straight-leg raises and range-of-motion exercises twice daily.
- Six months after total knee replacement, Mr. Palmer will return to his job as a police officer, able to perform usual job description as a policeman (able to walk two to three flights of stairs, participate in a chase on foot, and so forth).

Quality-of-life outcomes focus on key factors that affect someone's ability to enjoy life and achieve personal goals.

EXAMPLE QUALITY-OF-LIFE OUTCOMES

- Relates that pain is tolerable during key activities and sleep
- Absence of depression
- States that usual sleep patterns are back to normal
- Able to perform work and leisure activities

With some health problems, national health groups have identified key indicators to measure whether the patient's life is being positively impacted by the treatment plan. For example, pediatric asthma indicators include decreased emergency-room visits and improved attendance at school.

Discharge Outcomes and Discharge Planning

Identifying discharge outcomes and starting discharge planning early are the hallmarks of efficiency.[2] Today, the best discharge planning begins with outpatient education *before* admission and follows the patient throughout the continuum of care, including after discharge.

Discharge outcomes are written in broad terms, describing the level of assistance the person is likely to need at home (e.g., "Will be discharged home with care managed by wife and biweekly visits by home care nurse"). These statements may be followed by the indicators that describe the expected status of patient problems upon discharge (e.g., "Abdominal drains out," "Demonstrates wound care," and so forth). Box 4.3 shows a discharge planning questionnaire that helps you begin discharge planning early. Figure 4.5 shows a pathway for home care that's discussed with patients before they're admitted for heart surgery. You can see how this pathway helps patients to know what to expect when they leave the hospital.

Box 4.3	**Discharge Planning Questionnaire**

1. Is there a problem at home with any of the following?

	Yes	No	Possibly
● Heat	Yes	No	Possibly
● Hot/cold water	Yes	No	Possibly
● Electricity	Yes	No	Possibly
● Refrigeration	Yes	No	Possibly
● Cooking	Yes	No	Possibly
● Bathroom facilities	Yes	No	Possibly
● Stairs	Yes	No	Possibly
● Wheelchair accessibility	Yes	No	Possibly

2. Will the person require:

	Yes	No	Possibly
● Assistance with activities of daily living	Yes	No	Possibly
● Assistance with medications	Yes	No	Possibly
● Assistance with treatments	Yes	No	Possibly
● Additional teaching	Yes	No	Possibly
● Ongoing nursing assessment	Yes	No	Possibly
● Community resources or referrals	Yes	No	Possibly

3. Is necessary transportation available?   Yes   No   Possibly
4. How can the patient be reached by phone?
5. List available support systems (e.g., family, neighbors willing to help).

'AT HOME' PATH TO RECOVERY FROM CARDIAC SURGERY: THINGS TO DO EACH DAY				
Activity	*Health*	*Medications*	*Self-Care*	*Reasons to Call for More Information*
❑ Walk four times/day	Do each of the following items around the same time each day: ❑ Check your incisions ❑ Take your temperature by mouth (call if over 100°F)	❑ Take your medications as prescribed	❑ Keep your feet up while at rest ❑ Shower/bathe as instructed ❑ Practice reading food labels for fat intake, cholesterol, and sodium levels ❑ Eat healthy! Try new recipes	The nursing station phone number is (910) 716-6658. *Call your doctor if:* ❑ your heart rate (pulse) is less than 60 beats/minute or greater than 120 at rest, or ❑ you have severe chills, or ❑ unusual shortness of breath, or ❑ fever greater than 100°F (by mouth), or ❑ weight gain over 2 lb. in one day or 5 lb. in one week, or ❑ red or draining incisions, or ❑ chest pain, or ❑ if you have *any* questions or concerns
❑ Do exercises as prescribed ❑ Rest ❑ Limit visitors the first week or so (three to four people for 30 minutes/day) ❑ Resume sexual activities when ready ❑ After two weeks, help with light housework	❑ Check your pulse for one minute (normal: 60 to 120 beats/minute) ❑ Weigh yourself (call if you gain over 2 lb. in one day)	❑ Drink several glasses of water each day	❑ Wear stockings if ordered	

FIGURE 4.5   A home care pathway that's discussed with patients before they're admitted for heart surgery.

CASE MANAGEMENT

Case management—a method of care delivery that aims to improve outcomes and reduce costs through optimum use of resources—is an essential piece of *Planning*. Today, nurses in hospitals and communities are expected to recognize early when patients demonstrate problems that might require additional resources to achieve outcomes in a timely way. For instance, suppose your patient is a paraplegic who is having a routine cholecystectomy. This person is likely to have additional needs that an able-bodied person would not have. Early in the planning phase, ask, "Does this person have unusual or multiple health problems or disabilities?" If so, consider whether you should be asking your manager about getting additional resources, such as a case manager involved in the plan of care.

DECIDING WHICH PROBLEMS MUST BE RECORDED

Deciding which problems must be recorded is influenced by your understanding of the following:

- The person's overall health status and expected discharge outcomes.
- The expected length of contact with the patient (you have to be realistic about what problems can (and must) be tackled within the allotted time).
- The patient's perception of priorities. If the patient doesn't agree with your priorities, it's unlikely the plan will succeed.
- Whether there are standard plans that apply. For example, are there critical pathways, guidelines, protocols, procedures, or standard plans that address daily priorities for this particular patient's situation?

RULE **Follow policies and procedures for recording the plan of care carefully—these are designed to keep patients safe and to protect you from legal liability.** Patient records must communicate nurses' awareness of, and response to, all major care priorities. Some problems may not need to be recorded on the care plan because they are addressed in other parts of the record (e.g., Foley catheter care usually is addressed in policy and procedure manuals).

There are three main steps to determining which problems must be recorded.

1. Make a list of your patient's problems.
2. Decide which problems must be managed in order to achieve the overall outcomes of care.
3. Determine what documentation will guide how each problem will be managed (e.g., Doctors'orders? Following protocols? Critical pathway? Nurse-developed individualized plan? Patient self-manages?)

To communicate all major problems to the entire health care team, make sure that an up-to-date problem list with the status of current and past problems is in a prominent place on the patient record (Box 4.4).

Box 4.4   Example Multidisciplinary Problem List

Problem	Onset	Status 5/8/2011
Diabetes	2/11	See insulin and BS flow sheet. Gives own insulin
Anxiety/Coping	2/12	Sees APN for counseling once a week
Right knee replacement	4/10	Ambulatory, PT twice a week
Smoker (two packs/day)	1985	Down to one pack a day—smoking cessation counseling ongoing
Hypertension	2000	Stable—see med sheet
Asthma	1995	Stable—see current inhalers
Laminectomy	1996	Symptom free

RULE **Be sure that actual and potential problems that may impede progress toward outcome achievement are addressed in a prominent place somewhere on the patient record.** Doing this may require you to add a standard plan, modify a standard plan, or develop an individualized plan of your own.

CRITICAL THINKING AND CLINICAL REASONING EXERCISES

These exercises relate to the headings beginning with *Clinical Reasoning During Planning* and ending with *Deciding Which Problems Must Be Recorded.*

Example responses are provided at the end of the book (pages 206–207).

Part One: Setting Priorities For the Plan of Care

1. What are the four main purposes of the plan of care?
2. Using the memory-jog EASE, name the four components of a plan of care, giving an example of each.
3. List five factors that may influence how you set priorities.
4. If you had someone with the following problems, which problem would you need to treat immediately and why?

   a. Diarrhea

   b. Severe dyspnea

   c. Dehydration

5. What is the relationship between identifying expected discharge outcomes and setting priorities?

Part Two: Clarifying Expected Outcomes

1. What are the three main purposes of outcomes?
2. What four words are sometimes used interchangeably and usually mean the desired result of interventions?
3. Of the four terms you listed in number 2, which two terms are considered to be most specific?
4. a. If you identify an outcome and decide it's not within your qualifications to manage the problems that must be managed to achieve the outcome, what must you do?

   b. What must you do if it is within your qualifications?
5. What are your responsibilities during planning in relation to case management? (three sentences or less)

Part Three: Developing Outcome Statements

1. Why is it important to use measurable verbs when identifying outcomes? Give three examples of measurable verbs.
2. What are the five components of outcome statements?
3. Determine which of the following outcomes are written correctly. Identify what's wrong with the statements that are written incorrectly.

   a. Knows the four basic food groups by 1/4.

   b. Demonstrates how to use the walker unassisted by Saturday.

   c. Improves appetite by 11/5.

   d. Lists the equipment needed to change sterile dressings by 9/5.

   e. Walks independently in the hall the day after surgery.

   f. Understands the importance of maintaining a salt-free diet.

   g. Ambulates to the bathroom using her cane by 3/4.

   h. Loses 5 lb by 1/9.

   i. Feels less pain by Thursday.

4. For each diagnosis/problem, write an appropriate outcome:

   a. Impaired Oral Mucous Membrane related to poor oral hygiene

   b. Risk for Impaired Skin Integrity related to frequent diarrhea

   c. Impaired Communication related to inability to speak English

5. How does SMART help you remember key features of well-developed outcome and goals?

Part Four: Recognizing Affective, Cognitive, and Psychomotor Outcomes

Determine whether each of the following outcomes is in the affective, cognitive, or psychomotor domain. Use "a" for affective, "c" for cognitive, and "p" for psychomotor. (There may be more than one domain for each outcome.)

1. Demonstrates how to sterilize her baby's formula
2. Relates feelings concerning going home
3. Discusses the relationship between blood sugar levels and eating carbohydrates
4. Gives own insulin according to the results of morning blood sugar readings

DETERMINING NURSING INTERVENTIONS

Nursing interventions are actions performed by the nurse to:

1. Monitor patient health status and response to treatments.
2. Reduce risks.

3. Resolve, prevent, or manage problems.
4. Promote independence with activities of daily living (bathing and so forth).
5. Promote optimum sense of physical, psychological, and spiritual well-being.
6. Give patients the information they need to make informed decisions and be independent.

Nursing interventions are classified into two categories:

1. **Direct care interventions:** Actions performed through direct interaction with patients. Examples include helping someone out of bed and teaching someone about diabetes.
2. **Indirect care interventions:** Actions performed away from the patient but on behalf of the patient. These actions are aimed at managing the health care environment and promoting interdisciplinary collaboration. Some examples include monitoring results of laboratory studies and contacting a social worker.

Considering both direct and indirect interventions helps account for nurses' time. If you focus only on what the nurse does directly with the patient, you miss a lot of nursing time that's spent on other crucial nursing activities.

ASSESSMENT—MONITORING HEALTH STATUS AND RESPONSES TO CARE (SURVEILLANCE)

When planning care, it's important to consider what assessments need to be done to monitor status (nursing surveillance). Assessment may be planned specifically to detect or evaluate problems or to monitor responses to interventions. In fact, assessment is a part of every intervention. Your plan should reflect awareness of the need to assess the person at three key points:

1. Before you act, to be sure the action is safe and appropriate.
2. As you act, to monitor for adverse reactions.
3. After you act, to monitor the response.

PATIENT EDUCATION—EMPOWERING PATIENTS AND FAMILIES

Educating patients about their health and treatment plan, and motivating them to become involved in their own care, is the key to empowering them to become their own best advocate and caregiver. Patient education may be planned to enhance someone's knowledge about a specific problem (e.g., teaching about diabetes) or as part of an intervention to explain why it's being done (e.g., reinforcing the rationale for coughing and deep breathing as you're assisting the person to cough and breathe deeply). At every patient encounter, seize teaching opportunities. In complex situations, carefully plan what you're going to teach, and how you're going to teach it. Because teaching is a complex skill that includes paying attention to many different factors, the following guidelines are suggested to help you plan patient education.

Guidelines: Planning Patient Education

- Assess readiness to learn and previous knowledge before developing a teaching plan.
- Ask about preferred learning styles (e.g., a person who is a "reader" might want to read a pamphlet first, whereas someone who is a "doer" might want to handle equipment first). Adapt to the patient's preferred style rather than your own. (Download a handout on strategies for various learning styles at http://*www.AlfaroTeachSmart.com*.)
- Determine expected learning outcomes mutually with the patient, so that you both know what must be learned and mastered (e.g., "How would you feel about learning how to give an injection by Thursday?").
- Plan an environment that's conducive to learning, without interruptions.
- Identify active learning experiences. Use examples, simulations, games, and audiovisuals.
- Use simple terms, and teach basic concepts before moving on to more complex material.
- Plan learning experiences to build on successes.
- Encourage asking questions and verbalizing understanding of what is being taught (e.g., "I want you to feel free to ask questions no matter how insignificant you think they are. It's not easy learning something new. It is very important that you understand this.").
- Plan to pace learning. Don't give too much information at one time; progress at the person's learning pace.
- Allow time to discuss progress (e.g., to ask the person how he feels he's progressing) and to summarize what has been taught.
- Include significant others as indicated. See Box 4.5 for teaching those not fluent in English.

COUNSELING AND COACHING: HELPING PEOPLE MAKE INFORMED CHOICES

Counseling and coaching people to help them make needed changes in their lives—or to help them make choices about their health care—is another important nursing intervention that may be part of the plan. Counseling and coaching often include teaching and reinforcing key points in the plan of care (e.g., checking how diabetics are doing with following their diet and medications). Counseling and coaching also include exploring motivations and offering support during periods of adjustment to new circumstances. By using teaching and therapeutic communication techniques, you can

Box 4.5   **Educating Those Not Fluent in English**

1. Determine fluency for both speaking and reading English (some patients can read English better than speak it, and vice versa).
2. Get a translator for people not fluent in English.
3. Many teaching handouts are now available in other languages. You can download patient and caregiver handouts on common health issues in English and Spanish from *http://nursing.advanceweb.com/Clinical-Resources/Patient-Handouts/Patient-Caregiver-Handouts.aspx.*

offer valuable psychological and intellectual support, thereby reducing the stress associated with making choices about health care management. Helping to make informed decisions based on their own values and beliefs is an ethical responsibility of all nurses.

CONSULTING AND REFERRING: KEY TO MULTIDISCIPLINARY CARE

Making appropriate consultations and referrals is the cornerstone for multidisciplinary care delivery. For example, suppose you have someone who has trouble swallowing pills. You should be thinking, *I wonder if the pharmacist might know a better way to give medications (e.g., a liquid form).* If someone isn't eating because she dislikes hospital food, think about referring this problem to the dietitian so different meals can be served.

INDIVIDUALIZING INTERVENTIONS

The interventions you identify should aim to:

● Detect, prevent, and manage problems and risks.
● Promote optimum function, independence, and sense of well-being.
● Achieve the desired outcomes safely and efficiently.

Determining individualized interventions requires you to answer following questions, in context of each particular patient situation:

1. What can be done to prevent or minimize the risks or causes of this problem?
2. What can be done to manage the problem?
3. How can I tailor interventions to include patient preferences and meet the expected outcomes?

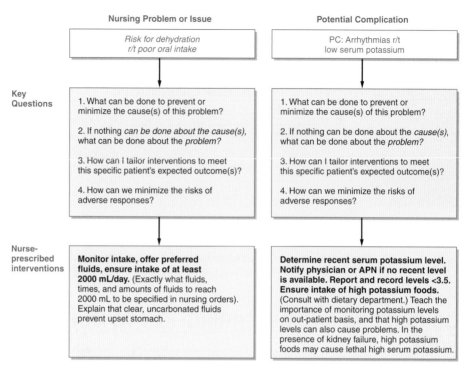

FIGURE 4.6 Example of how to determine nursing interventions.

4. How likely are we to get desired versus adverse responses to the interventions (and what can we do to reduce the risks and increase the likelihood of beneficial responses)?

5. What needs to be recorded about this intervention and how often should it be recorded?

Figure 4.6 maps the process of determining interventions. Figure 4.7 gives a worksheet to guide you when identifying specific interventions.

Evidence-Based Practice: Weigh Risks and Benefits

Evidence-based practice requires you to be aware of research that supports the use of the interventions you identify: If you're asked the question, "How do you know that this intervention works?" you should be able to answer by saying something like, "This is according to our protocols and procedures here in the hospital," or "This is recommended by national clinical practice guidelines." Or "Our textbook recommends this intervention." The point is that you should know the strength of the evidence that supports your interventions.

Before you choose an intervention, weigh the risks of causing harm against the probability of getting the desired results. To do this, answer the following questions:

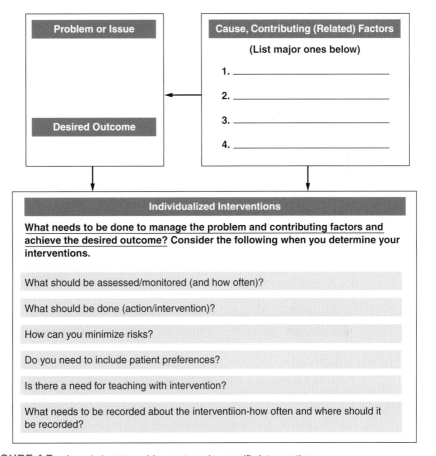

HOW TO DETERMINE SPECIFIC INTERVENTIONS

INSTRUCTIONS: Make sure interventions are *specific* to each situation by remembering PCO (Problem, Contributing factors, and Outcome). What needs to be done about the problem and contributing factors? How can you best achieve the outcome? Complete the boxes below. Use back of page as needed.

Problem or Issue

Desired Outcome

Cause, Contributing (Related) Factors

(List major ones below)

1. _____

2. _____

3. _____

4. _____

Individualized Interventions

What needs to be done to manage the problem and contributing factors and achieve the desired outcome? Consider the following when you determine your interventions.

What should be assessed/monitored (and how often)?

What should be done (action/intervention)?

How can you minimize risks?

Do you need to include patient preferences?

Is there a need for teaching with intervention?

What needs to be recorded about the interventiion-how often and where should it be recorded?

FIGURE 4.7   A worksheet to guide you to make specific interventions.

1. How reliable is the evidence that supports that the intervention(s) I plan to use is likely to work?
2. How likely are we to see the desired response in this particular patient and situation?
3. What is the worst thing that can happen if this intervention is performed, and how likely is it to happen?
4. What measures can we take to minimize the chances of causing harm?
5. What could happen if we do nothing about this problem or these risk factors?

Looking for Evidence-Based Care for the Elderly? Visit the Web site of The Hartford Institute for Geriatric Nursing, where you can find online resource for nurses in clinical and educational settings (http://consultgerirn.org/about/permissions/).

INDIVIDUALIZING NURSING ORDERS

The following guidelines help you individualize your nursing orders.

- Assess the person to determine a baseline of current signs, symptoms, and risk factors of the problem.
- Check for medical orders (e.g., medications, diet, activity, diagnostic studies, and so forth).
- If you use standard plans (e.g., critical path, protocol, preprinted or electronic plan), remember that you're responsible for:
  1. Detecting changes in patient status that may contraindicate using the plan.
  2. Using good judgment about which parts of the plans apply and which do not.
  3. Recognizing when problems aren't covered by the plan and finding other ways to address them e.g., some facilities have an additional page that can be placed on the record to address "out-of-the-box" situations).
  4. Adding unique patient requirements (e.g., walker) in appropriate places.

RULE To protect patients from errors and yourself from legal problems, use standard and electronic plans with a critical mind. Compare your patient's circumstances with the interventions listed in the standard or electronic plan. Decide what applies, what doesn't, and what's missing. Then modify (add, delete, or modify) interventions as indicated.

- Decide monitoring regimens for potential complications: What focus assessments need to be done to monitor the status of signs and symptoms? How often do assessments need to be recorded to spot trends?
- Identify interventions that prevent or minimize the underlying causes or risk factors of the problem and help achieve the expected outcome. For example, if you have "risk for injury related to chronic muscle weakness" with an outcome of "demonstrates safe ambulation with the use of a walker," tailor interventions to reflect that the person will be using a walker (e.g., have the person practice using the walker for ambulation in various circumstances, like going upstairs and downstairs and going to the bathroom).
- If you can't do anything about the causes or risk factors, decide what can be done about the problem. For example, if someone is terminally ill and has anxiety, you can't do anything about the fact that the person is going to die, but you can do something about the anxiety through counseling and therapeutic communication.

- Be sure the interventions are congruent with other therapies (e.g., allowing rest after physical therapy).
- Consider the person's preferences. Get input from the patient about how and when the interventions are performed. Individualize as much as possible.
- Determine the scientific rationale (evidence) for planned actions.
- Create opportunities for learning (e.g., explain rationale for all actions).
- Consult with other professionals when indicated (physician, APN, physical therapist).
- Before prescribing any actions:
  1. Weigh the risks and benefits of performing the actions.
  2. Make your orders specific: Keep in mind "see, do, teach, record" (i.e., what to assess [see], what to do, what to teach, and what to record).

EXAMPLE ORDERS FOR CARING FOR A SMOKER AFTER ABDOMINAL SURGERY

1. Assess breath sounds every 4 hours.
2. Help the person to perform coughing and breathing exercises with pillow and hand over incision every 4 hours.
3. Reinforce the importance of coughing and deep breathing.
4. Record breath sounds and sputum production once a shift and as needed.
5. Encourage the person to use current illness as a way to quit smoking.
6. Explore the person's knowledge on smoking cessation programs.

The following summarizes how to make sure your nursing orders are complete.

What to Include in Your Nursing Orders

Date: The date you write the order.

Verb: Action to be performed.

Subject: Who is to do it.

Descriptive phrase: How, when, where, how often, how long, or how much?

Signature: Be consistent in how you sign.

EXAMPLE

(Today's date) Assist patient to stand by the side of the bed for 10 minutes twice a day wearing her back brace. R. Alfaro-LeFevre, RN.

MAKING SURE THE PLAN IS ADEQUATELY RECORDED

The final phase of *Planning* is making sure that the plan is adequately recorded: You must be sure that all problems and risks that must be managed in order to achieve the overall outcomes of care are recorded somewhere in the patient record.

Forms for—and methods of—recording the plan of care are tailor-made to meet the needs of the nurses and patients in each unique setting. As you go from working in one place to another, remember the following rule.

> **RULE** **You are accountable for making sure your patient's plan meets each facility's specific standards.** Be certain that somewhere on the patient record, people can find evidence of the four main components of the plan of care (expected outcomes, actual and potential problems, specific interventions, evaluation/progress notes).

Box 4.6 gives a checklist to evaluate the plan of care to decide how it "measures up" compared with current standards. Box 4.7 summarizes key questions that need to be answered when developing a plan of care.

Box 4.6   **Checklist to Evaluate the Plan of Care**

1. Was the plan developed together with the patient and significant others and other key health care providers, as appropriate?
2. Have you addressed:
   - Actual and potential problems that must be managed to achieve the overall outcomes in a safe and timely way?
   - Problems that require individualized, not routine, nursing interventions?
3. If you identified problems that aren't on the plan of care, have you made sure that they are addressed somewhere in the patient's record (e.g., chest tube management might be addressed by physician's orders)?
4. Are the outcomes:
   - Derived from the diagnoses or problems?
   - Measurable?
   - Mutually formulated with the patient and other key players?
   - Realistic and attainable?
   - Written according to the rules (patient centered; measurable verbs; clear about who, what, when, how, and where)?
5. Do the nursing orders:
   - Include interventions that focus on controlling the underlying cause or risk factors of the problem (or, if that's not possible, treating the problem)?
   - Clearly direct interventions (addressing who, what, when, how, and how much)?
   - Incorporate use of resources and strengths?
   - Show the signature of the prescriber?
6. Does the plan:
   - Reflect current policies and practice standards?
   - Apply research and scientific principles?
   - Address developmental, psychosocial, spiritual, cultural, and biologic needs?
   - Include interventions for health promotion and teaching?
   - Provide for continuity (e.g., is it easily accessible, clear, and concise)?
   - Aim to reduce costs while promoting convenience and comfort?

| Box 4.7 | **Ten Key Questions Answered During *Planning*** |

1. **What major outcomes (observable beneficial results) do we expect to see in this particular person, family, or group when the plan of care is terminated?** Example: Three days after surgery, the person will be discharged, free from signs of infection, able to care for himself or herself.

2. **What problems, risks, or issues must be addressed to achieve the major outcomes?** Answering this question will help you set priorities. Study your problem list and narrow it down to those that *must* be addressed.

3. **What are the circumstances (what is the context)?** Consider things like who's involved (e.g., child, adult, group), whether the problems are acute or chronic, what factors are influencing the problems (e.g., when, where, and how the problems developed), and the patient's values, beliefs, and culture.

4. **What knowledge is required?** You must be clearly aware of individual patient circumstances, as addressed in #3 above. All the Knowledge CTIs listed in Chapter 1 are also required.

5. **How much room is there for error?** For instance, in which of the following cases do you think you have more room for error?

   ● You're trying to decide whether to give a healthy child a one-time dose of acetaminophen for heat rash without checking with the doctor.
   ● You have a child who's been sick for 3 days with a fever and the mother wants to know if she should continue giving acetaminophen without checking with the doctor.

   If you thought the first one above, you're right. In the second case, the symptoms have continued for 3 days without a diagnosis. If you make the mistake of continuing to give acetaminophen without checking with a physician, you might be masking symptoms of a problem requiring medical management.

6. **How much time do I/we have?** Be realistic about the amount of time you have with the patient. Accomplish what you can and consider referrals for follow-up care.

7. **What resources can help?** Human resources include clinical nurse educators, nursing faculty, preceptors, more experienced nurses, advance practice nurses, peers, librarians, and other health care professionals (pharmacists, nutritionists, physical therapists, physicians). The patient and family are also valuable resources (they know themselves best). Information resources include texts, articles, computer data bases and decision-support software; national practice guidelines; facility documents (e.g., guidelines, policies, procedures, assessment forms). Also consider financial resources, such as free community programs and services.

8. **Whose perspectives must be considered?** The most significant perspective to consider is that of the patient. Other important perspectives include those of key stakeholders (e.g., significant others, caregivers), relevant third parties (e.g., insurers), plus standards that apply to the patient's problems.

9. **What's influencing thinking?** Recognize personal values and beliefs, as well as biases and motivations of key stakeholders (e.g., families, insurance companies).

10. **What must be done to prevent, manage, or eliminate the problems, issues, and risks identified in #2 above?** Identify specific interventions aimed at achieving the outcomes; managing the problems, issues, and risks; and promoting function, independence, and well-being.

Addressing Patient Needs on Multidisciplinary Plans

Multidisciplinary approaches bring "the best of all worlds" together. Keep in mind, however, that as the nurse, you're the one at bedside the most. It's your job to stay focused on human responses—how the person is likely to respond as a whole to the plan—and to see that your patients' individual needs and desires are considered in the plan. Figures 4.8 and 4.9 show example care plans. Appendix A gives an example critical pathway that guides care for total knee replacement.

MULTIDISCIPLINARY REHABILITATION CARE PLAN

Patient Name: Robert Kirk	**Age:** 75 **Diet:** ADA	**Ht.** 5'7" **Wt.** 187 **Religion:** Cath.	**CARE REVIEW**
Primary Diagnosis:	**Allergies:** Sulfa		**Week of:** 7/14/13
R-THA 7/1/13	**Date Admitted:** 7/7/13 **Exp. Discharge:** 7/21/13		
Primary Physician: McGwire			

Primary Problems	Care Management	Status	Comments
Pain Management	Rehab Team	Current	Controlled. See flowsheet. Participating in therapy.
Impaired Mobility	Rehab Team	Current	Ambulation with walker with assistance 3 X day.
ADL Dysfunction	Rehab Team	Current	Minimal assistance.
Delayed wound healing	Wound Care Team	Current	(r) hip incision open 2 cm. Small amount pink drainage.

Co-Morbidities			
Parkinson's	Dr. Kostyo	Current	Stable with meds since 1995
Chronic A-fib with pacer (left side)	Dr. Foster	Current	On Coumadin since 2001. See anticoagulant flow sheet. Pacer rate set at 60. Rate controlled. Last checked pre-op 6/15
Glaucoma both eyes	Dr. Bell	Current	Stable with meds since 1999
Diabetes	Dr. Flynn	Current	Manages own BS and insulin

Discharge Planning			
Expected Discharge: 7/21/13 **Discharge outcome:** To home; primary caregiver wife; independent with walker; skilled care visits twice a week.	**Consults:** Case Manager: Home Health:	J. Knox VNA	**Other:** Anticoagulant reports to Dr. Foster

FIGURE 4.8   Example multidisciplinary plan of care. (© 2012 Terri Patterson, http://www.nursing consultation.com/)

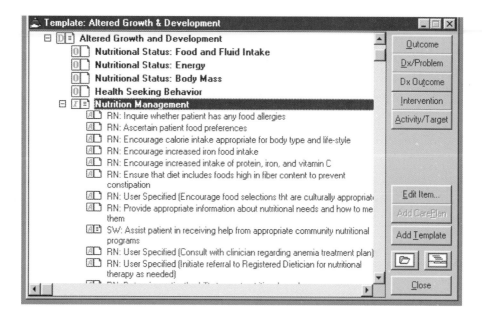

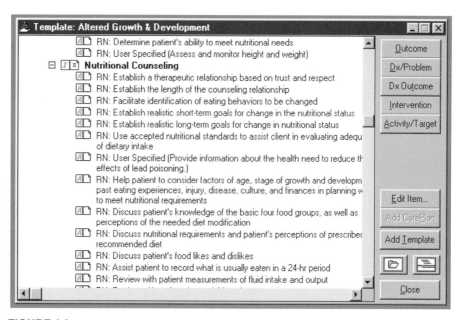

FIGURE 4.9   Two example screens from an electronic care plan. (Reproduced from CareManager software with permission of Egro Partners (http://*www.ergopartners.com*).)

CRITICAL THINKING AND CLINICAL REASONING EXERCISES

4.2   *These exercises relate to the headings beginning with Determining Interventions and ending with Making Sure the Plan Is Adequately Recorded*

Example responses are provided at the end of the book (pages 207–208).

Part One: Determining Interventions

1. What's the point of classifying interventions into direct and indirect interventions? (three sentences or less)
2. How do the words "see, do, teach, record" help you remember what you need to consider when determining interventions?
3. After you identify a problem, what two questions do you need to ask to determine interventions?
4. Explain how to weigh risks and benefits of interventions (five sentences or less).

Part Two: Individualizing Interventions Based on Problems and Outcomes

For each problem and outcome listed here, list some appropriate nursing interventions that might achieve the outcome.

1. Risk for pressure ulcers related to prescribed bed rest and loss of sensation in lower extremities
   Outcome: Maintains healthy intact skin with signs of adequate circulation
   Indicators: Absence of redness or irritation; management of risk factors recorded daily on skin protocol
   Nursing interventions:

2. Potential Complication: Atelectasis related to thoracic incision pain
   Outcome: Maintains clear lungs with absence of fever
   Indicators: Coughs effectively every 3 hours; lungs clear; relates pain does not inhibit breathing or coughing
   Nursing interventions:

3. Constipation related to medication side effects, insufficient exercise, and inadequate fluid and roughage intake as evidenced by no bowel movement in 4 days
   Outcome: Reports or demonstrates no constipation
   Indicators: Daily soft bowel movements; walks 20 minutes every day; drinks minimum of 2000 mL daily; demonstrates adequate roughage intake
   Nursing interventions:

Part Three: Monitoring to Detect Potential Complications

For each of the following problems, identify potential complications and determine a plan to monitor for the problems. (You may need to use additional resources, such as a medical–surgical textbook for this section.)

1. Intravenous infusion at 25 mL/h
   Potential complications:
   Plan for monitoring to detect potential complications:
2. Insulin-dependent diabetes
   Potential complications:
   Plan for monitoring to detect potential complications:
3. Foley catheter
   Potential complications:
   Plan for monitoring to detect potential complications:

Part Four: Ensuring the Plan Is Adequately Recorded

Using the memory-jog EASE, what four things do you need to check on the plan to be sure that the plan has been adequately recorded?

Try This on Your Own

With a peer, in a group, or in a personal journal:

1. Practice weighing risks and benefits and making decisions about interventions. Consider the interventions in the following situations and decide whether you would prescribe them and whether there is anything you could do to minimize the risks involved.
   a. Your neighbor calls at 10:00 PM and tells you her 9-year-old has chickenpox and generally is irritable and uncomfortable. She asks you if you think it would be okay to give her Children's Tylenol®. What would you tell her? What would you have told her if it were aspirin? Be sure to look up these drugs before answering.
   b. Mr. Evans is weak from being on bed rest. He reports being depressed because he's become so dependent on others. He's now allowed to go to the bathroom on his own and requests that he be allowed to do his daily hygiene unsupervised in the bathroom. You are concerned that he might tire in the bathroom. Would you prescribe for him to be allowed to do his morning care alone in the bathroom? If so, what would you do to minimize the risks?
   c. Your patient has a left chest tube and doesn't want to lie tilted to his left side because it's painful. Even though his right lung is compromised from previous disease process, he insists on being turned only to the right side. Would you allow him to turn only to his right side? If so, what would you do to minimize the risks?

2. Discuss the importance of viewing yourself as a risk manager, as addressed in the following article.

Midgley, M. Aumiller, L. and Moskowitz, M. (2011). Every Nurse is a Risk Manager retrieved January 27, 2011 from *http://ce.nurse.com/ce105-60/every-nurse-is-a-risk-manager/*

3. In a personal journal, with a peer, or in a group, discuss the implications of the following *Voices* and *Think About It* entries.

Voices

Building Relationships With Patients—Key to Good Nursing

Nursing is incredibly relational. We're invited into the most intimate moments of the lives of people who minutes before were strangers. We cannot truly care for people without knowing them, without knowing their values, fears, beliefs, relationships, and plans for their lives. So each day we are thrust deep into relational work that touches our own humanity in ways we often cannot anticipate. We need each other not just for support and understanding, but because the care requirements of patients are not limited to our shift or our day of assigned work. For us to do good work, to make a difference in the lives of our patients and their families, our work must be continuous, coordinated, and well communicated—shift-to-shift and nurse-to-nurse.[3]

—Gladys Campbell, RN, MSN

Nurses—Most Trusted Professionals

A Gallup survey shows that 84% of Americans rate nurses as "high" or "very high" for honesty and ethics. Since 1999, these surveys placed nurses at the top, except in 2001, when firefighters ranked first after the September 11 terrorist attacks. "The public's continued trust in nurses is well-placed, and reflects an appreciation for the many ways nurses provide expert care and advocacy,"[4]

—Karen Daley, American Nurses Association President

Think About It

Asking Negative Questions Helps You Set Priorities

When making decisions about what to record on the plan, ask yourself negative questions. Negative questions begin with, What could happen if I don't. For example, What could happen to this person if I don't address this problem on the plan of care? or What could happen if I don't report these signs and symptoms? Asking yourself these types of questions helps you focus on what's most important. If the answer is, "Not much can happen," you know the problem has a low priority. If the answer causes you concern, then you know the problem has a high priority.

Pain Management Promotes Healing

Pain management significantly improves your patient's ability to do what he needs to do to heal. The American Pain Society's quality improvement initiatives and Joint

Commission Standards stress that you must (1) promise patients that pain management will be a key part of the plan; (2) determine a way to monitor pain, treat it promptly, and evaluate the response; and (3) make information about analgesics and holistic interventions readily available for patients, families, and staff. For more information, go to http://www.thejointcommission.com, or http://www.ampainsoc. org—the Web site of the American Pain Society, a multidisciplinary educational and scientific organization dedicated to serving people in pain.

This Chapter and NCLEX

- Essential = Safety. When you see the word essential in the question (e.g., What essential actions must you plan?), the answer usually addresses something you must do to keep the patient safe.
- Expect questions on the monitoring (assessment) role related to procedures and drug administration. For example, What will you assess preprocedure, intraprocedure, and postprocedure? What will you assess before, during, and after drug administration?
- Pay attention to "time frame" words. For example, upon admission, prior to discharge, immediately prior to surgery, or just returned from (these determine the correct answer)
- Visualize and identify the outcomes (results) of each answer (is this desired?)
- Be prepared for many questions on setting priorities and delegating care (covered in the next chapter). Ask, if I can only do one thing for this patient what should it be? Remember, "Keep them breathing and keep them safe." When a question is unclear, think "safety."

Key Points

- Having a well-thought-out plan of care is the key to safety and efficiency and serves four main purposes: (1) Directs care and documentation; (2) Promotes communication and continuity of care; (3) Creates a record that can later be used for evaluation, research, and legal reasons; and (4) Provides documentation of health care needs for insurance purposes.
- Whether you develop your own plan or use a standard plan, you are responsible for following policies and procedures to make sure the plan is individualized.
- The memory-jog EASE helps you to remember the four main care plan components (Expected outcomes; Actual and potential problems; Specific interventions; Evaluation/ progress notes).
- Initial planning involves attending to urgent priorities and then determining expected outcomes of care. Outcomes for problems state what you expect to observe in the patient when the problems are resolved or controlled. Outcomes for interventions state the benefit you expect to observe in the patient after an intervention is performed (e.g., if you suction someone's tracheostomy, you expect that breath sounds will be clearer after suctioning). If you can't clearly identify the benefits you expect to see in the patient after nursing care, then you shouldn't be intervening.
- You determine the success of the plan by finding out if the patient achieved the expected outcomes. When writing outcomes, use measurable verbs. Outcomes may be written for affective, cognitive, or psychomotor domains.
- Patient records must communicate nurses' awareness of, and response to, all major care priorities; some problems may not need to be

recorded on the care plan because they are addressed in other parts of the record (e.g., Foley catheter care usually is addressed in policy and procedure manuals).

- The interventions you identify must be individualized to the patient and aim to: (1) Detect, prevent, and manage health problems and risks; (2) Promote optimum function, independence, and sense of well-being; and (3) Achieve the desired outcomes safely and efficiently.

- Evidence-based practice requires you to know the strength of the evidence that supports the use of the interventions you choose.

- Scan this chapter for important rules, maps, and diagrams throughout, then compare where you stand in relation to the expected learning outcomes in the chapter opener (page 129).

References

1. American Nurses Association. (2010). *Nursing: Scope and standards of practice* (2nd ed.). Silver Spring, MD: Nursesbooks.org.

2. National Health Service Institute for Innovation and Improvement. Quality and Service Improvement Tools: Discharge Planning. Retrieved January 16, 2012, from *http://www.institute.nhs.uk/quality_and_service_improvement_tools/quality_and_service_improvement_tools/discharge_planning.html*

3. Campbell, G. (1997). President's note. *AACN News, 14*(8), 2.

4. Daley, K. (2011). Nurses rank as most trusted profession yet again. Retrieved January 16, 2012, from http://news.nurse.com/article/20111213/NATIONAL02/112190001/1003

Chapter 5
Implementation

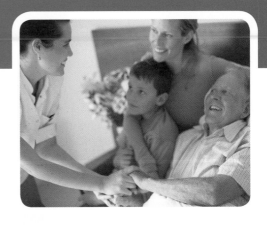

What's in This Chapter?

This chapter helps you understand your responsibilities related to *putting the plan into* action on a day-to-day basis. Here, you learn principles of giving and taking reports (hand-offs) and how to get organized, set priorities, and make the most of your time. You explore three topics you need to know for both NCLEX and clinical practice: (1) How do you prioritize care? (2) When is it appropriate to delegate care to others? (3) What steps must you take to ensure that you're delegating safely and effectively? You study your role as coordinator of care and gain insight into the importance of nursing surveillance (monitoring patient responses closely, observing for dangerous situations, catching errors early, and creating safety nets to keep patients safe). Finally, you learn key principles that help you chart effectively, whether you're using handwritten or electronic charting.

ANA Standards Related to This Chapter[1]

Standard 4   **Planning.** The registered nurse develops a plan that prescribes strategies and alternatives to attain expected outcomes.

Standard 5   **Implementation.** The registered nurse implements the identified plan.

Standard 5a   The registered nurse coordinates care delivery.

Standard 5b   Health Teaching and Health Promotion: The registered nurse employs strategies to promote health and a safe environment.

Standard 6   **Evaluation.** The nurse evaluates progress toward attainment of outcomes.

Critical Thinking and Clinical Reasoning Exercises

Exercises 5.1   Giving and Taking Reports (Hand-offs), When and How To Delegate; Using Standard Plans and Identifying Care Variances; Performing Interventions

Exercises 5.2   Principles of Effective Charting

Expected Learning Outcomes

After studying this chapter, you should be able to:

1. Explain how *Implementation* is related to both *Planning* and *Evaluation*.
2. Discuss how you'll give and take hand-off reports the next time you're in the clinical setting.
3. Identify strategies for getting organized and setting priorities the next time you're in the clinical setting.
4. Delegate safely and effectively by applying delegation principles as described in this chapter.
5. Address your role in relation to coordinating care, nursing surveillance, preventing care omissions and adverse outcomes, and building safety nets.
6. Explain your role related to case management and variances in care.
7. Describe how to weigh risks and benefits to reduce the likelihood of harm from an intervention.
8. Describe how the words "assess, re-assess, revise, record" apply to performing interventions.
9. Explain the six main purposes of charting.
10. Discuss the characteristics of effective charting systems.
11. Apply principles of effective charting.
12. Chart effectively, applying principles of effective charting and following facility policies and procedures.
13. Keep your patient's plan up-to-date.
14. Evaluate your work days to determine changes that can reduce your stress and improve your performance.

IMPLEMENTATION: PUTTING THE PLAN INTO ACTION

In this chapter, you learn how to put the plan into action in a safe, effective, and organized way—a way that increases the likelihood of getting the results you need while preventing errors and other undesirable results.

Remember the following diagram from Chapter 1 that shows how *Implementation*—putting the plan into action—is like "a bridge" between *Planning* and *Evaluation*.

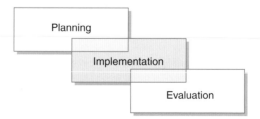

Implementation is linked to both *Planning* and *Evaluation* for two main reasons:

1. *Planning* guides care during *Implementation*.
2. As you implement care, you begin early evaluation, making changes as needed. You don't wait for the formal evaluation phase to determine how your patients are responding to care.

This chapter focuses on the following main activities.

IMPLEMENTATION

☐ Giving and taking reports (hand-offs)
☐ Setting daily priorities
☐ Delegating appropriately
☐ Coordinating care
☐ Surveillance (monitoring responses; preventing errors, omissions, and adverse outcomes)
☐ Building safety nets
☐ Performing interventions
☐ Charting effectively
☐ Keeping the plan up-to-date
☐ Evaluating your day

RULE **Your ability to communicate** (listen, speak, and write effectively) with patients, families, unlicensed workers, and other professionals makes the difference between competent, efficient care and care that's sloppy, unprofessional, and prone to errors.

Implementation is challenging because that's where "the action is," with many dynamic variables affecting your performance. It also requires you to put all five steps of the nursing process together while "thinking in action" to make quick decisions. It requires you to:

1. Assess patients to be sure their status hasn't changed and interventions are still appropriate.
2. Recognize when problems or issues have changed.
3. Plan before you act.
4. Perform nursing actions (interventions).
5. Evaluate responses carefully, and revise your approach as indicated.

RULE **Remember "assess, re-assess, revise, record":** *Assess* patients before you perform nursing actions. *Re-assess* them to determine their responses after you perform nursing actions. *Revise* your approach as indicated. Record patient responses and any changes you made in the plan.

Having discussed the importance of applying all five phases of the nursing process during *Implementation* in a "seamless" way, let's go on to address key things you'll need to do on a daily basis in the clinical setting.

GIVING AND TAKING REPORTS (HAND-OFFS)

In most cases, your clinical day begins and ends with hand-off change-of-shift reports. Hand-offs also occur whenever care passes from one nurse's hands to another (e.g., when a patient is transferred from one unit to another). Hand-off tools are also often completed before calling physicians to report signs and symptoms that you're concerned about.

Using standard hand-off tools does three things:

1. Helps you get organized
2. Prevents omissions of key information that must be communicated
3. Promotes dialogue and critical thinking between caregivers

Whenever you start a new position, ask for policies and procedures for hand-offs and follow them closely. Don't rely on memory. Because what you say during hand-offs and how you say it influences quality of care that your patient receives, the following gives guidelines for giving reports (hand-offs).

Guidelines: Giving Reports (Hand-Offs)

● **Follow policies and procedures for giving hand-offs.**
● **Be specific.** Avoid vague terms.

> **EXAMPLE OF BEING SPECIFIC DURING HAND-OFFS**
> **Right:** "Mrs. Wu has had an increase in her respiratory rate to 32 per minute. Her heart rate is up to 122, and her temperature is 101°F."
> **Wrong:** "Mrs. Wu seems to be having respiratory difficulty."
> **Right:** "I gave Mrs. Wu 8 mg of morphine IM at 5:10 PM for incision pain."
> **Wrong:** "I gave Mrs. Wu a pain med around 5 PM."

● **If you make an inference, back it up with evidence.** (e.g., "Seems upset with her husband—crying and saying that he doesn't support her.")
● **Describe the status of all invasive lines** (e.g., IV lines, Foley catheters, nasogastric tubes).
● **Stress abnormal findings** (e.g., abnormal breath sounds or vital signs) and variations from routines. (e.g., "This patient *won't* be medicated before surgery.")
● **Ask for clarification when needed.** Apply read back and repeat back rules as indicated.

Figure 5.1 gives an example hand-off tool that uses the SBAR format. You can also download evidence-based strategies and tools from a free hand-off tool kit

SBAR (Situation, Background, Assessment, Recommendation)*

NOTE: Pronounced S-BAR and first used by the military to improve the effectiveness of communication between care givers, the SBAR approach is recommended by patient safety experts. SBAR forms vary depending on purpose and setting. Some places use SBAR for giving hand-off situations (when one nurse transfers patient care to another). Some places use SBAR forms like the one below for calling physicians about a problem.

→ **Have the chart in hand before you make the phone call, and be sure you can readily communicate all of the following information.**

S **SITUATION:** Have the chart in hand before you make the phone call, and be sure you can readily communicate all the following: Briefly state the issue or problem: what it is, when it happened (or how it started) and how severe it is. Give the signs and symptoms that cause you concern.

B **BACKGROUND:** Give the date of admission and current medical diagnoses. Determine the pertinent medical history and give a brief synopsis of the treatment to date (eg, medications; oxygen use; nasogastric tube; IVs, code status).

A **ASSESSMENT:** Give most recent vital signs and any changes in the following:

- ☐ Mental status – neuro signs
- ☐ Respirations
- ☐ Pulse – skin color
- ☐ Comfort – Pain
- ☐ GI status (nausea-vomiting-diarrhea, distention)
- ☐ Urine Output
- ☐ Bleeding-Drainage
- ☐ Other: _____

R **RECOMMENDATION:** State what you think should be done. For example:

- ☐ Come see the patient now
- ☐ Get a consultation
- ☐ Get additional studies (eg, CXR, ABG, EKG, CBC, other)
- ☐ Transfer the patient to ICU
- ☐ If the patient doesn't improve
- ☐ How frequent do you want vital signs.
- ☐ If there's no improvement, by when do you want us to call you?

*Data from: Haig, K, Sutton, S. and Whittington, J. (2006). SBAR: A Shared Mental Model for Improving Communication Between Clinicians. *Journal of Quality and Patient Safety*, *32*(3), 167–175. Available: http://www.jcipatientsafety.org/fpfd/psp/SBAR.pdf

Source: R. Alfaro-LeFevre Handouts © 2007–2013 www.AlfaroTeachSmart.com

FIGURE 5.1   SBAR, a common hand-off tool.

to enhance performance and patient safety at *http://www.ahrq.gov/qual/teamstepps/* and *http://www.aorn.org/PracticeResources/ToolKits/PatientHandOffToolKit/*.

SETTING DAILY PRIORITIES

Setting priorities during *Implementation* requires applying the same principles of setting priorities addressed in the section on "Attending to Urgent Priorities" in Chapter 4. Take a few moments to review that section now (pages 131–132).

The following section gives additional strategies to help you set daily priorities when you care for more than one patient.

Guidelines: Prioritizing Care for Several Patients

- **Make initial quick rounds** of your patients, briefly checking the "big picture" of how they're doing (try to do this before you go to get a hand-off or review patient records). **Rationale:** This helps you to identify problems requiring immediate attention and helps you to connect the actual patients with what you hear during the hand-off or read in patient records.
- **Immediately after hand-offs,** verify critical information such as IV infusions, operation of equipment, and so forth. **Rationale:** Verifying information you received during report is a "safety net" that helps you identify discrepancies between what you heard and what is actually happening.
- **Do quick priority assessments and identify urgent problems** (those posing an immediate threat to the patient, e.g., chest pain or a disconnected IV line) and take appropriate action (e.g., get help if needed). **Rationale:** Attending to urgent problems takes priority over taking time to analyze all the patient's problems.
- **List your patients' major problems** in relation to the expected outcomes for the day and answer the following questions:
  1. Which problems must be resolved today, and what happens if I wait until later?
  2. Which problems must I monitor today, and what could happen if I don't monitor them?
  3. To achieve the overall outcomes of care, which are the problems, issues, or risks that must be resolved or managed today?

  Rationale: You can only do so much in a day. Answering these questions helps you decide what must be done *today*.

> **RULE** **Partner with patients to set priorities—set mutual goals for the day.** Start by asking patients their most important goals for the day. For example, "Tell me three main things you want to accomplish today," or "What are the most important things you want me to help you with?" This sets the tone for mutual goal setting. It helps you to avoid making assumptions about what's important to your patients and also helps you to identify assumptions your patients may have made (e.g., they may have unrealistic expectations).

- **Determine the interventions that must be done to prevent, resolve, or manage the problems on your problem list.** List these interventions along with routine tasks such as baths and meals. **Rationale:** This helps you to get a big picture of the tasks of the day, which helps you to answer questions such as, What must be done first? and How can I make the best use of my time? For example, you may give a routine bath to promote hygiene and, at the same time, discuss problems with coping.

- **Decide what things the patient or significant others can do on their own, what things to delegate to others, and what things you must do yourself** (when and how to delegate is addressed in the next section). **Rationale**: Encouraging patients and families to be as independent as possible helps them take charge of their own care. Often, patients and families don't know what they are or aren't expected to do for themselves. Using less qualified help appropriately allows you to spend more time accomplishing tasks that require the expertise of a registered nurse.

- **Make a personal worksheet for getting things done for the day and refer to it frequently.** Be sure to consider the daily routine of the unit (e.g., when meals are served). **Rationale**: You'll experience many distractions during the course of the day and should not rely on memory. Although the daily routine of the unit shouldn't dictate your activities, it's vital to consider it when setting the schedule. For example, it's frustrating to both nurses and patients when meals arrive during baths or patients are called to physical therapy at inconvenient times.

WHEN AND HOW TO DELEGATE

Nurses today are increasingly accountable for delegating certain aspects of care to other workers. Delegating safely and effectively is a skill that takes in-depth critical thinking and grows with on-the-job experience. You also need to understand principles of delegation to answer NCLEX questions.

Delegation is defined as *transferring to a competent individual the authority to perform a selected task in a selected situation while retaining accountability for results*[2]—you are accountable for the outcomes of care you delegate. For example, suppose you delegate care of a child to Jane, an unlicensed worker. Jane tells the mother to watch the child while she's at lunch. If the mother leaves the room and something happens to the child, YOU are accountable.

> **RULE** **When you delegate care, check the results yourself.** Checking the results of care you delegate keeps patients safe, protects you from legal liability, and encourages good care (workers are more likely to do a good job when they know you will be checking the *results*).

Study Box 5.1 that addresses the five rights and four steps of delegation. Then study Figures 5.2 and 5.3 that map the critical thinking you need to do before delegating care.

Box 5.1   Five Rights and Four Steps of Delegation

Five Rights
Delegate (1) the right task, (2) in the right situation (3) to the right worker, (4) with the right direction and communication, and (5) the right teaching, supervision, and evaluation.

Four Steps
1. **Assess and Plan**: Consider the patient, the task, and worker competencies to make a plan for what tasks you will assign to whom (see Figures 5.2 and 5.3).
2. **Communicate**: Give clear, concise, complete directions about what must done, how it must be done, what needs reporting, and when to touch base with you (verify that worker understands directions).
3. **Ensure Surveillance and Supervision**: Monitor the patient and worker performance as frequently as needed based on the above.
4. **Evaluate and Give Feedback**: Evaluate the effectiveness of the delegation by assessing patient response yourself. Decide whether you need to make changes in the patient's plan of care or how the worker is completing the task. Evaluate worker's performance and give teaching and feedback as needed (this helps worker improve skills and ultimately frees you for other important work).

Source: American Nurses Association and National Council of State Boards of Nursing. (2006). *Joint Statement on Delegation*, Accessed January 27, 2012 from *https://www.ncsbn.org/Joint_statement.pdf*

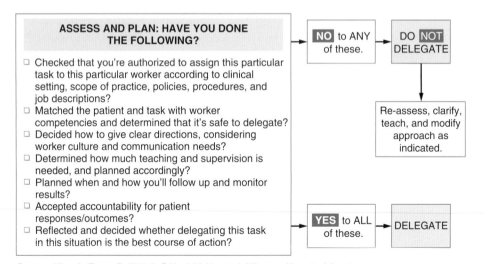

Source: Alfaro-LeFevre, R. (2011). Critical thinking tool: When and how to delegate.
No use without permission.

FIGURE 5.2 Assessment and planning you need to do before you delegate. (Source: Alfaro-LeFevre, R. (2011). *Critical Thinking Tool: When and How to Delegate*. No use without permission. http://*www.AlfaroTeachSmart.com*)

MATCH THE PATIENT AND TASK WITH WORKER COMPETENCIES	
PATIENT AND TASK ➡	**WORKER COMPETENCIES**
☐ Patient stable? Needs assessed? ☐ Included in decision-making? ☐ Environment SAFE? Task still indicated? ☐ Outcome of the task for this patient is reasonably predictable? ☐ Directions for task are unchanging and easy to follow? ☐ Does NOT require complex or frequent assessment by you? **NOTE:** The above relates to unlicensed workers. LPNs and RNs may perform more complex tasks, depending on SBN rules and regulations. Tasks requiring the nursing process or RN assessment and judgment may be delegated to RNs ONLY.	☐ Task occurs frequently in daily care and is within workers' scope of practice, skills, and job description? ☐ Passed competency tests if needed? ☐ Expresses familiarity with related policies and procedures? ☐ Asks questions and for help as needed? ☐ Clarifies (repeats back) what must be done, what to report, and when to touch base with you? ☐ Expresses comfort with this task in this specific patient situation? ☐ Plans for patient safety, privacy, comfort, and cultural needs?

Source: Alfaro-LeFevre, R. (2011). Critical thinking tool: When and how to delegate. No use without permission.

FIGURE 5.3   Matching the patient and task to worker competencies before you delegate. (Source: Alfaro-LeFevre, R. (2011). *Critical thinking tool: When and how to delegate.* No use without permission. http://*www.AlfaroTeachSmart.com*)

COORDINATING CARE

National practice standards stress that nurses are responsible for coordinating care during *Implementation* and for documenting coordination of care.[1] As the nurse, you are with patients the most, so pay attention to the overall care patients receive. Reflect on their treatment schedule and how it's affecting them. Encourage patients to let you know if there are things that they would like to be organized differently (e.g., patients who are "morning people" should have physical therapy treatments in the morning). Be sure to record how overall care can best be coordinated on the plan of care.

RULE   When coordinating care, remember the importance of thinking ahead, thinking in action, and thinking back (reflecting) during *Implementation*.[3] **Think ahead** (be proactive—anticipate what might happen and how you can be prepared). **Think in action** (pay attention to what's going on in your head as you "think on your feet," gathering and putting information together). **Think back** (reflect on your thinking to decide what you can learn from what happened, what influenced your thinking, and what you can do better next time—this usually requires dialogue with others or journaling to make your thoughts explicit).

SURVEILLANCE—PREVENTING ERRORS AND OMISSIONS— CREATING SAFETY NETS

Nursing surveillance—paying careful attention to what's happening to your patients at the point of care—is a critical part of *Implementation*. It includes all of the following:

1. Monitoring patient status and responses to care
2. Monitoring for error or risk-prone processes
3. Checking for care omissions
4. Making corrections and building safety nets to reduce the incidences of numbers 1–3 above.

RULE   Keep patients safe during *Implementation* by preventing errors and omissions and building safety nets. Monitor closely for error-prone situations. Find ways to catch possible errors and omissions early. Collaborate as needed to create safety nets for all important care situations (e.g., ask someone to double check your math on a complex drug calculation).

How to Identify, Interrupt, and Correct Errors

Hennenman et al. identify that nurses use the following strategies to identify, interrupt, and correct errors.[4]

- **Error identification strategies:** knowing the patient, knowing the "players," knowing the plan of care, surveillance, knowing policy/procedure, double-checking, using systematic processes, and questioning.
- **Error interruption strategies:** offering help, clarifying, and verbally interrupting.
- **Error correction strategies:** persevering, being physically present, reviewing or confirming the plan of care, offering options, referencing standards or experts, and involving another nurse or physician.

Figure 5.4 shows how monitoring for dangerous situations promotes early correction of problems and keeps patients safe.

Keeping an Open Mind

Monitoring patient responses requires assessing with an open mind. Too often nurses are so influenced by the hand-off report that they forget to dig a little deeper into patient situations, as noted in the following example.

EXAMPLE

The Importance of Assessing With an Open Mind. During report, Jodi, the evening nurse, was told, "Mrs. Ross is a difficult patient—she won't ambulate." Later, when Jodi went to give Mrs. Ross her medications, she asked if there was something that was causing her to be so tired. Mrs. Ross responded that she hadn't slept well in weeks because she had just found out her daughter had breast cancer and was afraid she might lose her. This was important information that hadn't been offered before. Jodi then was able to talk with Mrs. Ross about her fears and offer a positive outlook by explaining that breast cancer, when detected early, has a good prognosis. By later that evening, Mrs. Ross was ambulating and talking about how eager she was to go home.

> ### RULE
> **Use every patient encounter as an opportunity to observe mental and physical status and to empower patients to care for themselves (through teaching, coaching, and so forth).** For example, if you're helping someone bathe, assess skin status (by observing the entire body) and mental status (by using therapeutic communication techniques). This is also an opportunity to teach good skin care.

POTENTIAL DANGEROUS SITUATIONS

TECHNICAL ISSUES	HUMAN ISSUES	SYSTEM FAILURE ISSUES
Examples: alarms not working, broken equipment, computer issues	**Examples:** poor attention, knowledge, or skill; fatigue; failure to follow policies and procedures	**Examples:** poor staffing; poor training; room design that makes it difficult for nurses to maintain infection control; poorly designed workflow. Technical and human issues on left may also be the result of system failure issues.

NURSING SURVEILLANCE AND SAFETY NETS
Monitoring for the above dangerous situations; interrupting and correcting error-prone situations; building safety nets to catch mistakes before they happen.

☐ Early detection, prevention, and correction of errors.
☐ Reporting of organizational failure issues.

RESULTS
☐ **No adverse patient outcome** (or reduction in severity of adverse patient outcome)
☐ **Correction of system failure issues**—improved organization safety measures

FIGURE 5.4   How monitoring for dangerous situations promotes early correction of problems and keeps patients safe. (**Source**: © 2010 http://*www.AlfaroTeachSmart*.com. No use without permission.)

PERFORMING NURSING INTERVENTIONS

Performing interventions entails getting prepared, performing interventions, determining responses, and making necessary changes. Chapter 4 addresses how to determine *individualized* interventions. This section addresses how to *implement* interventions.

Be Proactive—Promote Safety, Comfort, and Efficiency

Adequate preparation before performing an intervention makes the difference between risky, haphazard care that taxes both you and the patient and efficient, safe care that promotes comfort and gets results. Before you perform an intervention, ask the following questions:

● Am I qualified and is it prudent?
● What might I need?
● What could go wrong, what can I do to prevent it from happening, and am I prepared to deal with it, if it does happen?
● Is my patient ready and is the intervention still appropriate?
● What can I do to make this easier?
● Are there any policies and procedures I need to check?

RULE Always get patients' agreement before moving forward with interventions.

IMPLEMENTATION AND EVIDENCE-BASED PRACTICE

National practice standards stress the need to implement the plan of care using evidence-based interventions. As a thought-oriented, rather than task-oriented, nurse, be sure you can answer the question, "What evidence supports that these interventions are likely to work?" In some cases, you'll have several research studies cited in policies and procedures to support planned interventions. In others, you may only know that the interventions are recommended in a reliable text. Either way, don't settle for the answer, "This is how we always do it." Be sure you understand the strength of the evidence behind your interventions.

Having addressed the importance of knowing the strength of the evidence that support your interventions, the following guidelines address other important thinking you need to do before performing interventions.

Guidelines: Preparing to Perform Interventions

● **Review the plan and be sure you know the rationale and principles** behind the interventions. If you don't know the principles and rationale, you won't be able to adapt the procedure if you need to, and you may not even recognize if the intervention is no longer indicated.

- **Decide whether you're competent and qualified** to perform the interventions (if not, seek help).
- **Find out whether there are relevant facility procedures, protocols, guidelines, or standards** that address how you should perform the interventions.
- **Assess the patient's current status** and decide whether the interventions still are appropriate and whether he or she agrees to the intervention.

RULE **Always use two unique identifiers to be sure you have the right patient.** For example, ask the person his name and birth date and also check the identification bracelet to make sure it matches.

- **Predict possible outcomes to your interventions.** Get a picture of what you're going to do, and think about what might come up, what could go wrong, and what you'll do about it.
  1. Weigh risks and benefits of intervening versus doing nothing.
  2. Identify ways to reduce risks of harm to the patient and yourself.
  3. Determine how to promote comfort and reduce patient stress (e.g., if someone is expected to sit for a long time, get a comfortable chair and offer distractions).
- **Obtain the required resources** (e.g., equipment, personnel) and make sure you planned enough time and an environment conducive to performing the interventions.
- **Involve patients and significant others.** Explain what's to be done, why it's going to be done, and how long it will take. Encourage them to voice questions, suggestions, or concerns.

RULE **Before performing any intervention, ask yourself,** Am I clear about what I'm going to do, how I'm going to do it, and *why* it's indicated for this *specific* person?

Clinical Reasoning—What to Do When Things Go Wrong

Even when you're fully prepared, you may not get the desired response to your interventions. Let's look at what to do if you don't get the desired response, if the problem shows no improvement, or if the situation is aggravated by what you did.

If you don't get the desired response, a red flag that says "something's wrong" should go up in your mind. Stop and ask some key questions:

1. **Did I perform the interventions correctly?** For example, if you suctioned someone who sounded congested and there was no mucus, did you have enough suction and did you direct your tubing the way you needed to?
2. **Is the diagnosis correct, or has the problem or its cause changed?** For example, suppose you were caring for a woman with tachycardia, and her heart rate didn't come down as you expected after giving a medication to slow the

heart rate. Your next questions should be something like, Could there be something else causing or contributing to the tachycardia? Could anxiety, fever, or a respiratory problem be causing this fast heart rate?

3. **Are there other interventions that may complement this intervention, increasing its effectiveness?** For example, a backrub and talking with someone who's anxious is likely to enhance the effect of an anti-anxiety agent.
4. **What could I be missing?** Should I get a second opinion?
5. **If you make a mistake,** take immediate steps to minimize patient harm; then follow policies and procedures for reporting errors.

> **RULE** **Monitor patient responses carefully as you carry out nursing actions.** If you don't get the desired response, find out *why* and make corrections before continuing to act.

STANDARD PLANS AND CARE VARIANCES

If you use standard plans to guide your patient's care, you'll find that they set priorities for you on a day-by-day basis—that is, it does unless you identify a care variance. A care variance is said to have occurred when a patient hasn't achieved outcomes by the time frame noted on standard plan. For example, suppose the plan you are using states "By the second day after surgery, the patient will be out of bed in a chair three times a day," but you decide your patient isn't well enough to be out of bed three times a day. This discrepancy between what your patient is able to do and what the plan states he *should* be able to do is called care variance.

Identifying care variances should trigger you to do additional assessments to determine whether the delay is justified or whether actions need to be taken to improve the likelihood of achieving the outcome.

> **RULE** **When using standard plans, don't assume your patient is ready to progress as planned: look for care variances.** If you identify a care variance, consider whether you need to contact additional professional resources for in-depth assessment and treatment.

ETHICAL AND LEGAL CONCERNS

Having addressed the importance of assuring patient privacy, let's look at some other ethical and legal concerns related to outcomes. Ethically—and in some cases, legally—you're responsible for emotional outcomes of your interventions, as well as physical outcomes. For example, in some states, it's against the law to tell people they have AIDS over the phone. You must tell them in person and provide counseling and support. Here's another example: Suppose your patient is having a facial tumor removed, and the standard plan is to give a pamphlet with graphic pictures of reconstructive surgery. As a prudent nurse, you must anticipate this response, stay with the person, and provide support.

CRITICAL THINKING AND CLINICAL REASONING EXERCISES

5.1 Giving and Taking Reports (Hand-Offs); When and How to Delegate; Using Standard Plans and Identifying Care Variances; Performing Interventions

Example responses are provided at the end of the book (pages 208–209).

Part One: Giving and Taking Reports (Hand-Offs)

1. What three main things does using standard hand-off tools accomplish?
2. When are the two main times that hand-off tools are used?

Part Two: When and How to Delegate

1. Fill in the blanks below using the following words: situation, authority, competent, accountability, selected

   According to the ANA and the National Council of State Boards of Nurses, delegation is defined as transferring to a _____ individual the _____ to perform a _____ task in a selected _____ while retaining _____ for results.

2. Applying the five rights of delegation means delegating the right _____ to the right _____ with the right direction and _____, and the right _____, _____, and evaluation.

3. Before delegating care, you must match the patient and the task to the workers capabilities. (a) What does this mean? (b) Why must you do it?

4. One of the most important things in delegation is monitoring patient outcomes and worker performance. How do you do this and why?

5. Suppose that one of the many tasks that you have to do today is getting a 60-year-old woman who has had a routine cholecystectomy out of bed for the first time.

   a. Would you delegate this task to an unlicensed worker?

   b. Why or why not?

Part Three: Using Standard Plans and Identifying Care Variances

Answer the following questions, using three to five sentences.

1. How do you assess a patient for a care variance?
2. What would you do if you identified a care variance and why?

3. What can happen to the patient if you miss the fact that your patient is demonstrating a care variance?
4. What can happen to you if you miss the fact that your patient is demonstrating a care variance?

Part Four: Performing Interventions

What do the following have to do with performing nursing interventions?
1. Assess and re-assess
2. Nursing surveillance
3. Errors and omissions
4. Being proactive
5. Comfort, safety, and efficiency
6. Getting patient agreement

Try This on Your Own

1. Learn more about teamwork, communication, and rapid response systems. Download theTeamSTEPPS Rapid Response Systems Guide from *http://www.ahrq.gov/teamsteppstools/rrs/index.html*.
2. In a personal journal, with a peer, or in a group, discuss the implications of the following *Voices* and *Think About It* entries.

Voices

Issues Contributing to Care Omissions

Evidence points to the omission of required nursing care as a pervasive problem in acute care hospitals. Nine areas of care omission in nursing have been identified including ambulation, turning, delayed or missed feedings, patient teaching, discharge planning, emotional support, hygiene, intake and output documentation, and surveillance. Reasons cited for missed care include too few staff, increased complexity of care, poor use of staff resources, increased time required for nursing interventions, poor teamwork, ineffective delegation, habits of cutting corners, and denial of the issue and impact.[5]

—*Researchers Bittner, Gravlin, Hansten, and Kalish*

Include Nursing Assistants and Patients in Hand-Offs

I REALLY want to stress the importance of RNs and nursing assistants (NAs) doing shift hand-offs *together* with patients. Shift report is the perfect time for giving effective initial direction and for collaborative RN and NA planning (the off-going NAs can be answering call bells). Assignments must reflect good delegation and supervision principles. Doing bedside reports ensures that patients and families are included in planning from the start.

—*Ruth Hansten, RN, MBA, PhD, FACHE (Email communication)*

Stressed Out? Remember, First Things First!

When I'm under stress, I take the advice of flight attendants: Put your own oxygen mask on first.

—*Randy Pausch, Author of The Last Lecture*

Do Your Best and Leave the Rest

Too many of us burn out trying to do it all. I can't do all "little things" that I'd like to do. On the way home from work, I remind myself, "Do your best and leave the rest."

—*Jeanne Regn, RN, Staff Nurse (personal communication)*

Think About It

Using Huddles Improves Teamwork and Efficiency

In sports, teams gather together in a huddle to motivate or celebrate. In health care, getting the team together for a few minutes to address major goals or issues for the day gets everyone on the same page and promotes teamwork. Huddles should be <10 minutes and can be held at the beginning of the shift or whenever significant changes in work flow arise. Getting the team in a huddle to discuss what's happening and make adjustments that improve work flow aids both patients and staff. Patients benefit from better use of resources. Staff benefit because they know their needs will be communicated and feel like a team who is playing the same game for the same reason: Improved patient care quality and efficiency.

Preparing for Report (Shift Hand-Off)

Preparing for shift hand-off—learning about patient problems, looking up common treatments, reading charts, and getting to the unit early—reduces your stress and improves your efficiency. Too often, there's little time for reading charts and looking up management of common problems during the course of the day. When you make time to prepare yourself for the day, you feel more confident, are more competent, and can begin giving care in a timely way.

Promoting Health: Exercise Caution

There are many opportunities to promote health by stressing the need to exercise every day. However, be sure to teach the "Ask Your Doctor First" rule. Those starting an exercise regimen should check with their primary care provider to be sure it's safe and appropriate for them.

Caring Means More Than Being Nice

Caring means more than being friendly and nice. Patients do value this type of caring. But, what they want even more are knowledgeable, competent nurses who closely monitor their care. They want nurses who carefully double-check care management and advocate when something is wrong or could be improved.

Act FAST When You Suspect a Stroke

The window of opportunity to avoid permanent brain damage from stroke is short (3 hours). Use the memory-jog FAST to guide assessment and action when you suspect your patient has a stroke:

F–Facial weakness—can the person smile? Has their mouth or eye drooped?
A–Arm weakness—can the person raise both arms?
S–Speech problems—can the person speak clearly and understand what you say?
T–Time to call 911

Source: Adapted from several online documents.

CHARTING

After you give nursing care, your next priority should be charting assessments, interventions, and patient responses to care. Two reasons for this are:

1. **Charting what you've observed and done often jogs your memory about something *else* you need to assess or do.** For example, you may be charting an abdominal assessment and realize that you forgot to check whether the nasogastric tube equipment is functioning properly.
2. **You're likely to be more accurate and thorough when your memory is fresh.**

Six Purposes of Charting

The main purposes of your charting are to:

1. **Communicate care** to other health care professionals who need to be able to find out what you did and how the person is doing.
2. **Help you and others to identify patterns** of responses and changes in status (you identify patterns by reviewing charting over time).
3. **Ensure evidence-based care.** Most charting systems prompt you to record information and interventions that evidence has shown must be done within specific time frames (e.g., giving an antibiotic within a certain amount of time of doing blood cultures).
4. **Provide a basis for evaluation,** research, and improvement of care quality.

5. **Create a legal document** that later may be used in court to evaluate the type of care rendered. Your records can be your best friend or worst enemy. The best defense that you assessed your patient or performed interventions is that you recorded what you did on the patient record.
6. **Supply validation** for re-imbursement from Medicare, Medicaid, and other insurance companies for the cost of care. The saying goes, "if it's not recorded, they won't pay."

RULE **You're accountable for following policies and procedures for documenting on the patient record.** Failure to follow these may jeopardize patient care and put you at risk for being accused of giving substandard care.

This section focuses on charting during *Implementation*. Additional information on charting during *Assessment* can be found in Chapter 2, in the section on *Reporting and Recording* on pages 81–84.

Various Ways of Charting

There are various ways of charting, as charting systems seem to be changing almost as quickly as you can say "computer." Depending on where you work, you may use any of—or a combination of—the following charting methods (these are often incorporated into electronic health records).

- **Source-oriented charting:** Each discipline charts in it's own particular place on the record (e.g., nurses chart only on nursing records).
- **Multidisciplinary charting:** All health care professionals—nurses, physicians, nutritionists, etc.—chart on the same record.
- **Flowsheet charting:** You use specific sheets or computer fields to enter focus assessments to track the status of specific patient conditions.
- **Charting by exception (CBE):** You refer to unit standards, policies, and protocols in the patient record, charting narrative notes only when the patient's data change or care deviates from the norm.
- **Addendum sheet charting:** You use supplemental records, adding separate sheets for each type of situation (e.g., discharge summary sheets, teaching sheets).

Whatever charting method you use, the goal is the same—to have charting that is:

- Accurate, factual, and complete
- Organized and standardized
- Timely and easily accessible (it should be easy for you to chart in a timely way and easy for others to find the information they need)

Figures 5.5, 5.6, and 5.7 give examples of various types of charting.

FLOWSHEET: ABDOMINAL ASSESSMENT*						
Date/Time	8/8 7am	8/8 7pm	8/9 7am	8/9 7pm	8/10 7am	8/10 7pm
Abdominal girth Signs/symptoms	48" Pain at +3 feels bloated	52" NC	48" Pain at +2 Bloated	46" Pain at +2 Bloated	44" Pain free Bloated but less so	
Bowel sounds	Absent	NC	Distant	Distant	↑ activity	
N/G drainage	Small amt green	NC	NC	NC	NC	
Bowel movement	None	NC	NC	Passed gas	↑ passing gas	
RN Initials	RAL	DL	RAL	DL	RAL	

* If there is no change in finding, chart "nc."

FIGURE 5.5   Example flowsheet charting.

PRINCIPLES OF EFFECTIVE CHARTING

Because you're likely to work with a broad range of charting methods—from hand-written to electronic charting—it's important for you to learn universal principles of effective charting. Applying the following principles will help you adapt from one charting method to another. It will also help you to answer questions related to documentation on NCLEX.

1. When others read your charting, they should see evidence of the following:
    ● **Initial and ongoing assessments:** What did you observe when you first encountered the patient and at subsequent encounters (especially before and after interventions)?
    ● **Status of patient problems:** What are the patient's current signs and symptoms?
    ● **Interventions and nursing care performed:** What did you do to meet the person's needs?
    ● **Patient response (outcomes of care):** What results did you observe?

NORMAL INFANT ASSESSMENT PARAMETERS

NOTE: Normal findings for head-to-toe assessment are listed below. If your assessment of the infant yields data that match listed normal assessment parameters, place a check mark($\sqrt{}$) and your initials to the right of the box. If assessment findings *vary* from listed normals, place an asterisk (*) in the box, mark your initials to the right of the box, and explain variance in the nurse's notes. Do NOT initial unless you have carefully assessed each area and compared it with the normal parameters.

HEAD: Soft, level, fontanelles; sutures approximated; normal hair; no infections, lice, lesions, cuts or bruises. ☐

EENT: PERLA. Focuses appropriately. Responds appropriately to voices. No ear pulling or drainage; TM's pearly and external canals clear. Nares patent without discharge. Mouth and throat without lesions. Moist, pink mucous membranes. Trachea midline and neck supple. Gag reflex present; normal swallowing & sucking. No lymphadenopathy. ☐

RESP: Rate normal for age. Breath sounds vesicular throughout lungs and bronchial over major airways without adventitious sounds. No nasal flaring or retractions. No cough. ☐

CARDIOVASCULAR: Regular heart rate within normal range for age. No extra heart sounds. Bilateral peripheral pulses satisfactory. No cyanosis (lips and nail beds). No edema, rapid capillary refill. ☐

SKIN: Skin warm, dry, & intact. Normal turgor. No red areas, rashes, bruises, lesions, lumps, or lacerations. Moist, pink mucous membranes. ☐

GI: Abdomen soft and non-tender with bowel sounds in all 4 quadrants. No hernias. tolerates diet. No nausea or vomiting. BM's normal (pattern, consistency, color). ☐

(See page two for neurological, orthopedic, and urologic parameters)

Nurse Signature: _____ Date: _____ Time: _____

FIGURE 5.6 Example nursing data base showing normal infant assessment parameters, with directions for charting by exception (CBE).

ANTICOAGULANT TEACHING RECORD

Name: John Roch   **Age:** 75   **Diagnosis:** Chronic Atrial Fib

Primary care manager at home: Self   **Drug name:** Coumadin

	Teaching Done			Outcome Met
Note: Encourage patient to refer to patient information handouts, rather than trying to memorize. Give patient a blank copy of this page on first day of teaching and a copy of completed form at discharge. **Expected outcomes:** By _7/11_ , you should be able to:				
1. Produce a folder of teaching handouts to keep for reference, and identify where this folder will be kept at home.	7/7 RA	7/9 DL	——	7/9 DL
2. Explain why anticoagulant medication and close monitoring of anticoagulant blood level is essential.	7/7 RA	7/9 DL	——	7/9 DL
3. Relate when and where to go for first appointment for blood work (PT, INR)	7/7 RA	7/9 DL		7/9 DL
4. Describe: ❏ drug, action, and how dose will be determined ❏ drugs that may affect dosage (eg, ASA, NSAIDS, Vit K) ❏ foods that may affect dosage and must be avoided ❏ how to assess for unusual bleeding ❏ how to avoid injury or bruising (eg, using electric razor) ❏ how to treat cuts and bruise to minimize bleeding and injury ❏ the importance of reporting persistent headache	7/7 RA	7/9 DL	——	7/9 DL
5. Explain the need to report: ❏ unusual bleeding or bruising. ❏ to all doctors and dentists that anticoagulant is being taken.	7/7 RA	7/7 DL	——	7/9 DL
6. Carry a medic alert card or jewelry stating anticoagulant name.	7/7 RA	7/9 DL		

Comments/Progress Notes:

7/7 Teaching initiated pre-op. Uses handouts well   RA
7/9 Waiting for medic alert ID. DL

Patient Signature _____   Discharge Nurse's Signature _____

FIGURE 5.7   Example addendum sheet charting showing patient education.

- **Any specific attention given to safety or undesirable outcomes:** What did you do to ensure patient safety? If you didn't get the desired response in the patient, what did you do?
- **The person's ability to manage care needs after discharge:** What did you observe and do in relation to the likelihood that the patient is able to manage his own care?

2. **Effective charting systems should:**
   - **Be tailored to the types of problems frequently seen** in the patient population of the facility—they should direct nurses to chart key aspects of care.
   - **Reflect use of the nursing process and be legally sound.**
   - **Discourage double documentation** (charting the same thing in two different places). **Increase the quality of patient records** while reducing the amount of time spent on charting.
   - **Be designed so that key patient information (e.g., assessments and interventions) is easily retrievable,** thereby facilitating communication, evaluation, research, and quality improvement.

Avoiding Dumping Syndrome With Electronic Charting

When using electronic charting, it's important to avoid "dumping syndrome." Dumping syndrome is the tendency to dump information into a computer and forget about it: data go from your brain to the computer, and there they sit, lost to the brain.

Find ways to reflect on your charting, either through printouts or cues in the system. If you don't make time to look for patterns, consider the big picture, and think about what you might be missing—you're not thinking critically. You're simply dumping data into a computer.

Learning to Chart Effectively

Charting effectively requires knowledge, experience, and application of principles of effective charting. As you improve your ability to perform assessments and discriminate between normal and abnormal findings, your charting will improve.

It's also important to do two things:

1. Practice using whatever type of charting you'll be using before you go to the clinical setting.
2. Read charts to learn from actual situations. As you read the charts, ask yourself questions like, What are the diagnoses? Where's the evidence that the diagnoses exist? What are they doing to treat them? and How is this person responding?

Guidelines: Charting During Implementation

- **To identify omissions and changes in patient status,** chart as soon as possible, following policies and procedures carefully.
- **Reflect on what you chart,** asking questions like, Am I missing anything? and How does what I'm charting compare with what the people before me charted? This helps you recognize changes in status early.

- **Record important actions immediately** to be sure that others know the action has been completed.
- **Record all variations from the norm** (e.g., abnormalities in respiration, circulation, mental status, or behavior) and any actions taken related to the abnormalities (e.g., if you reported the abnormality or if you intervened in some way).
- **Be precise.** Your notes should give a description and timeline for sequence of events, answering the questions of what happened and when, how, and where it happened.
- **Focus on significant problems or events that communicate *what's different*** about this person today. For example, don't record "went to the bathroom unassisted" unless this is unusual.
- **Stick to the facts.** Avoid judgmental language.

> **(EXAMPLE)**
>
> Right: "Shouting, 'Everyone had better stay away from me, or I'm going to hit someone.' "
> Wrong: "Angry and aggressive."

- **Be specific.** Don't use vague terms.

> **(EXAMPLE)**
>
> Right: "Abdominal dressing has a 6 inch circle of light pink drainage."
> Wrong: "Noted moderate amount of drainage on abdominal dressing."

- **Be concise, yet as descriptive as you can be.** You don't have to write complete sentences. Use adjectives and accepted abbreviations to give a good picture of activities and observations. For example, "OOB to chair for a half hour—c/o slight dizziness on standing up but moved well."

RULE Check "Do Not Use" lists and use only accepted abbreviations.

- **Sign your name consistently** using your first initial, last name, and credentials after each entry that you complete (e.g., "R. Alfaro-LeFevre, RN").
- **If you forget to chart something, record it as soon as you can,** following procedures for making late entries.

> **(EXAMPLE)**
>
> 5/17 3:00 PM, Late entry: Stool was positive for blood at 10 AM this morning. Notified Dr. Eyler—R. Alfaro-LeFevre, RN.

- **If you make a mistake on a chart, correct it according to facility policies.** Do not hide mistakes.
- **Record refusal to follow prescribed regimen,** as well as any actions you took. For example: "Refuses to go to physical therapy. Says it 'doesn't do any good.' Notified Dr. Frazier and Rochelle Hutton in physical therapy."

Charting Memory-Jogs

The following memory-jogs can help you remember some common approaches to charting narrative notes.

- **AIR-A (Assessment, Intervention, Response, Action).** Chart the assessment data you observe, the interventions performed, the patient's response to interventions, and any actions you took based on the response.
- **DARA (Data, Action, Response, Action).** This has the same meaning as the above.
- **SOAP, SOAPIE (Subjective data, Objective data, Analysis, Plan; Subjective data, Objective data, Analysis, Plan, Intervention, Evaluation).** Chart the subjective and objective data you collected, your analysis of what the data indicate (your conclusion), and the plan. With SOAPIE, you also add the intervention(s) you performed and the evaluation (patient response) after the intervention(s) were performed.

KEEPING THE PLAN UP-TO-DATE AND EVALUATING YOUR DAY

While the next chapter gives details on comprehensive *Evaluation*, let's complete this chapter by addressing the importance of keeping the plan up-to-date and evaluating your workday. Remember that ANA performance standards specifically address two issues related to evaluation during implementation[1]:

- **Quality of care:** The nurse systematically evaluates the quality and effectiveness of nursing practice.
- **Performance appraisal:** The nurse evaluates (her or his) own nursing practice in relation to professional practice standards and relevant statutes and regulations.

The following are the types of questions you should be asking on a daily basis to make sure the plan of care is kept up-to-date.

Determining If the Plan of Care Is Up-to-Date

- Does your patient still exhibit the problems identified on the plan?
- Are there risks that need to be addressed?
- Does your patient have problems that *aren't* addressed on the plan of care but *should* be?
- Are the expected outcomes still realistic?
- Are the interventions still relevant?

Box 5.2 lists questions to ask yourself to evaluate your workday.

Box 5.2	Evaluating Your Workday

Ask yourself:
- How has the day gone in general?
- How would my patients evaluate me in relation to meeting their specific needs?
- Have I identified my learning needs (should I be looking up information or getting advice from a more experienced nurse)?
- Have I been organized and able to set priorities well?
- What factors are influencing how I set priorities and organize my day?
- Could I be doing more? Am I trying to do too much?
- Am I acting in a collegial way? Have I been clear and specific when delegating actions and communicating with others?
- Am I including patients and families as partners in care?
- What changes should I make tomorrow?

CRITICAL THINKING AND CLINICAL REASONING EXERCISES

5.2   Principles of Effective Charting

Example responses are provided at the end of the book (page 210).

1. What are the six main purposes of charting?
2. Give two main reasons why you should chart as soon as possible after giving nursing care.
3. Get a piece of paper and write a note that records the following events using the mnemonic AIR-A.
   A patient calls you into the room and tells you that she feels like she's choking on mucus but is afraid to cough because of incision pain. You help her to get in a better position and then teach her to splint the incision with a pillow. She coughs up a gray mucus plug and thanks you for your help. You listen to her lungs, and they sound clear. You emphasize the importance of reporting pain so that it can be managed to promote her ability to cough to clear lungs.
4. What's wrong with the following two excerpts from nurses' notes?
   a. 5/8 Patient is difficult and uncooperative. R. Alfaro-LeFevre, RN.
   b. 5/8 Patient seems confused. R. Alfaro-LeFevre, RN.
5. Give three reasons why always following charting policies and procedures is of utmost importance.

6. Pretend you wrote and signed the nurse's note below on the wrong chart. Correct it using an accepted method for correcting charting errors.

   5/8 N/G tube draining light green drainage.

7. How does "dumping syndrome" relate to electronic health records?

Try This on Your Own

1. **Fall and injury prevention continues to be a challenge in all aspects of care.** According to the research, unintentional falls are the most common cause of nonfatal injuries for people older than 65 years in the United States. Up to 32% of people in the community over 65 fall each year. Females fall more frequently than males in this age group. Fall-related injuries are the most common cause of accidental death in those over the age of 65. Learn more about research on falls by going to www.ahrq.gov and searching for "fall and injury prevention."

2. In a personal journal, with a peer, or in a group, discuss the implications of the following.

Voices

We Don't Make Charting Rules, But We MUST Follow Them

All patients admitted with a diagnosis of pneumonia need to have an antibiotic within a specific time frame, or Medicare won't pay us. Check once, check twice, check three times. If your patient has CHF (congestive heart failure), be sure you record that you gave him CHF discharge instructions, even if he only has a *history* of CHF or we won't get paid then either!!! YES!!! YES!!! Patient care is always the most important part of nursing! We just have to "play the game" as well. In the end, it means better patient care!

—*Posting on a Staff Development Listserv*

Think About It

Evidence-Based Practice Challenges Assumptions About Restraints

Many people assume that restraining agitated patients protects them from harm. On the contrary, evidence shows that physical and chemical (drug induced) restraints may actually cause serious injuries, emotional and physical problems, and costly complications.[6] To learn more, read *Safety Without Restraints: A New Practice Standard for Safe Care* posted at http://www.health.state.mn.us/divs/fpc/safety.htm.

Evidence-Based Protocols Guide Care

As we continue to track treatment and outcome data, protocols and critical pathways guide care. For example, if you have *pneumonia*, you'll probably receive a specific antibiotic that's been proven to give the best results and most cost-effective approach.

Ten Rights of Medication Administration

To promote high-quality, safe care, apply the "ten rights" of drug administration: right patient, drug, time, dose, route, reason, follow up assessment, documentation, patient education, right to refuse.

This Chapter and NCLEX

- Expect case scenario questions that ask you about delegation (what should you delegate, to whom, and when?) and prioritization (what should you do *first?*). Review the section on *How and When to Delegate.*
- When asked questions on performing interventions, remember "Assess, Re-assess, Revise, Record."
- Expect pharmacology questions that address patients rights related to drug administration—remember the "ten rights" (right patient; right drug; right time; right dose; right route; right reason; right follow up assessment; right documentation; patient's right to refuse, and be educated about medications).
- Remember patient safety standards, especially the importance of using two unique identifiers to identify the patient before performing interventions.
- To answer questions about what to chart on the patient record, apply the content under *Principles of Effective Charting—Learning to Chart Effectively—Guidelines: Charting During Implementation—Charting Memory-Jogs*

Key Points

- Whereas the last chapter focused on developing and recording an *initial* plan of care, this chapter addresses the clinical reasoning you need to do to *put the plan into* action in a safe and effective way.
- The following key *Implementation* activities are stressed in this chapter: Setting Daily Priorities; Delegating Appropriately; Coordinating Care; Surveillance (monitoring patient responses; preventing errors, omissions, and adverse outcomes); Building Safety Nets; Performing Interventions; Charting Effectively; Keeping the Plan Up-to-date; Evaluating Your Day.
- Human responses are unpredictable. Monitor them carefully—be flexible and change approaches as needed in a timely way. Record changes you make in the chart and on the plan of care.
- Knowing how to communicate effectively and build positive relationships with patients, families, and coworkers is key to *Implementation*.
- When you put the plan into action, use an active, open mind—you should be constantly

assessing and re-assessing both patient responses and your own performance.

- Knowing how to delegate effectively is a key required competency of all registered nurses and important for passing NCLEX.
- Learning to chart effectively comes with practice and experience. *Always* follow policies and procedures for communicating care (charting and giving hand-off reports).
- Avoid the dumping syndrome (dumping data into a computer and forgetting about it). Unless you reflect on what you chart—to identify patterns, consider the big picture, and identify things you may have missed—you're not thinking critically.

- ANA performance standards address the need to evaluate the quality and effectiveness of nursing practice. This means evaluating nursing practice in general and also evaluating your own performance in relation to professional practice standards and relevant statutes and regulations.
- An important part of *Implementation* is evaluating how your own day went and determining ways you can be more organized and less stressed.
- Scan this chapter for important rules, maps, and diagrams highlighted throughout, then compare where you stand in relation to the expected learning outcomes in the chapter opener (page 160).

References

1. American Nurses Association. (2010). *Nursing: Scope and standards of practice* (2nd ed.). Silver Spring, MD: Nursesbooks.org.
2. American Nurses Association and National Council of State Boards of Nursing. (2006). *Joint Statement on Delegation*, Accessed January 27, 2012 from *https://www.ncsbn.org/Joint_statement.pdf*
3. Alfaro-LeFevre, R. (2012). *Critical thinking indicators: Evidence-based version*. Retrieved January 27, 2012, from *http://www.alfaroteachsmart.com/NewCTIReq.htm*
4. Henneman, E., Gawlinski, A., Blank, F., Henneman, P., Jordan, D., & McKenzie, J. (2010). Strategies to Identify, Interrupt, and Correct Medical Errors: Theoretical Framework. *American Journal of Critical Care, 19*(6), 500–509.
5. Bittner, N., Gravlin, G., Hansten, R., & Kalish., B. (2011). Unraveling care omissions. *Journal of Nursing Administration, 41*(12), 510–512.
6. Minnesota Health Department. *Safety without restraints: A new practice standard for safe care.* Retrieved September 1, 2012 from *http://www.health.state.mn.us/divs/fpc/safety.htm*

Chapter 6
Evaluation

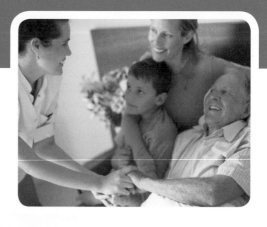

What's in This Chapter?

Whereas Chapter 5 stressed the importance of doing *ongoing evaluation*—assessing and re-assessing patients to monitor initial responses to care during *Implementation*—here you learn how to do a comprehensive evaluation that helps you decide whether the patient is ready for discharge. You also explore your responsibilities related to research, quality improvement (QI), and evidence-based practice (EBP), as addressed by Quality and Safety Education for Nurses (QSEN) competencies and Institute of Medicine (IOM) competencies.[1-3] Finally, you gain insight into the importance of improving quality by studying outcomes (results), process (how you got the results), and structure (the setting or environment) in which you got the results.

ANA Standards Related to This Chapter

Standard 7   **Evaluation.** The registered nurse evaluates progress toward attainment of outcomes.[4]

Critical Thinking and Clinical Reasoning Exercises

Exercises 6.1   Determining Outcome Achievement, Identifying Variables Affecting Achievement, and Deciding Whether to Discharge the Patient

Exercises 6.2   Quality Improvement, Research and Evidence-Based Practice, Examining Errors, Infections, and Injuries

Expected Learning Outcomes

After studying this chapter, you should be able to:

1. Describe how to do a comprehensive evaluation of an individual plan of care.
2. Explain the relationship between *Evaluation* and the other phases of nursing process, including the special relationship between *Planning* and *Evaluation*.
3. Address the relationship between outcomes and deciding whether to terminate or modify the plan of care.
4. Determine where your patients stand in relation to outcome achievement.
5. Evaluate your patients to decide whether they're ready for discharge or whether you need to continue or revise the plan.
6. Discuss the relationship between patient outcomes and how health care systems interact with one another.
7. Explain why it's important to do all three types of evaluation studies—outcome, process, and structure—to improve care quality.
8. Describe your four main responsibilities related to QI and research.
9. Explain the relationship between nursing research and EBP.
10. Give six key questions you need to answer before you can apply research to practice.
11. Participate in research and EBP studies to improve care quality.
12. Apply principles of reflective practice to learn from challenging situations.

EVALUATION: KEY TO EXCELLENCE IN NURSING

Evaluation—careful, deliberate, appraisal of various aspects of patient care—is the key to excellence in nursing. It makes the difference between care practices that are risky and error prone and care practices that are safe, efficient, and constantly improving.

This chapter first examines how to evaluate the care of individual patients, and then it discusses what you need to know about QI—studies that aim to improve outcomes by evaluating the effectiveness, efficiency, and safety of human performance and health care delivery processes.

EVALUATION AND THE OTHER PHASES OF NURSING PROCESS

While *Evaluation* involves examining what happened during all the nursing process phases, there's a significant relationship between *Evaluation* and *Planning*. This relationship is illustrated by the shaded boxes at the top of the next page.

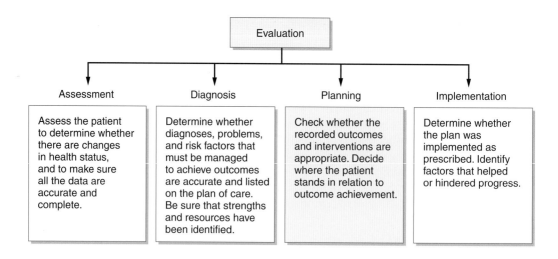

EVALUATING AN INDIVIDUAL PLAN OF CARE

Evaluating how a plan has worked for a particular patient involves the following:

- Determining where the patient stands in relation to outcome achievement
- Identifying variables (factors) that affected outcome achievement
- Deciding whether to discharge the patient or continue or change the plan

Let's begin by looking at guidelines for evaluating outcome achievement.

Guidelines: Determining Outcome Achievement

- Assess the patient to determine current health status and readiness to test for outcome achievement.
- List the outcomes set forth in *Planning*.

EXAMPLE

Will walk unassisted with crutches the length of the hall by 7/3.

- Compare what the person is able to do in relation to the outcomes.

  EXAMPLE

  Can walk unassisted the length of the hall, but becomes unsteady toward the end of the hall.

- Answer the following questions:
  1. Has the patient completely achieved the outcomes?
  2. Has the patient only partially achieved the outcomes?
  3. Has the patient not achieved the outcomes at all?
- Record your findings on the patient record according to policies and procedures (usually on progress notes or plan of care).

Identifying Variables (Factors) Affecting Outcome Achievement

Identifying the variables (factors) affecting outcome achievement means deciding what things influenced your patient's ability to get the desired results. This requires doing an in-depth patient assessment, analyzing the patient's record, and involving the patient, family, and caregivers to answer questions like the following:

- Was the patient involved in setting daily goals?
- To what level was the patient included in determining outcomes and fine-tuning interventions?
- Were the outcomes and interventions realistic and appropriate for this person?
- Were the interventions consistently implemented as prescribed?
- Were problems and risks identified and managed *early?*
- What's the patient's opinion concerning outcome achievement and the plan of care?
- What factors impeded progress?
- What factors enhanced progress?
- Have we applied the most up-to-date EBP strategies?

Deciding Whether to Discharge the Patient

The final step in evaluating how an individual's plan of care has worked is deciding whether to discharge the patient, to continue the plan as is, or to modify it to incorporate approaches that are more likely to succeed.

- **Continue the plan** if the person hasn't achieved outcomes, but you simply need more time.
- **Change the plan** when the person hasn't achieved outcomes and you've identified new problems or risks that need managing, or if you've identified more efficient interventions.
- **Terminate the plan and discharge the person** if he has achieved outcomes, has no new problems or risk factors that must be managed, and is able to manage his own care.

  Box 6.1 gives steps for terminating the plan.

| Box 6.1 | **Steps for Terminating the Plan of Care** |

1. Ask the patient and family how health care will be managed at home.
2. Give verbal and written instructions for:
   ● Treatments, medications, activities, diet
   ● What signs and symptoms to report (when to call the doctor)
   ● How to reach relevant community resources
3. Ask the person to repeat (or show you) what has been learned (notes or instructions may be used to jog memory).
4. If the person (or caregiver) demonstrates knowledge of how to manage health care at home, terminate the plan and discharge the patient according to facility policy.

CRITICAL AND CLINICAL REASONING EXERCISES

 Determining Outcome Achievement, Identifying Variables Affecting Achievement, and Deciding Whether to Discharge the Patient

Example responses are provided at the end of the book (page 210).

Part One: Determining Outcome Achievement, Identifying Variables Affecting Achievement

For each number below, compare the outcome criteria with the listed observable patient data. Put an "A" in the margin if the outcome has been achieved. Put a "P" if the outcome has only been partially met. Put an "N" if the outcome has not been met.

1. **Outcome:** Will demonstrate self-injection of insulin using aseptic technique.
   Observable data: Able to give actual injection well, but I had to first point out she had contaminated the needle without noticing it.

2. **Outcome:** Will demonstrate safe walking with crutches, including climbing and descending stairs.
   Observable data: Demonstrates ability to use crutches for walking, climbing, and descending without problems.

3. **Outcome:** Will relate the effect of increased exercise on insulin demand.
   Observable data: States that insulin demand is not affected by increased exercise.

4. **Outcome:** Will maintain skin free from signs of irritation.
   Observable data: Skin is intact with some reddened areas noted on both elbows.

5. **Outcome:** Will list the major signs and symptoms of infection.
   Observable data: Lists pain, swelling, and drainage.

Part Two: Deciding Whether to Discharge the Patient

How do you know whether to terminate, continue, or change the plan? (three sentences)

Try This on Your Own

Learn how nurses impact on patient outcomes. Explore the web page of National Database of Nursing Quality Indicators (NDNQI)®, a repository for nursing-sensitive indicators. NDNQI® is a national nursing data base that provides quarterly and annual reporting of structure, process, and outcome indicators to evaluate nursing care at the unit level. Linkages between nurse staffing levels and patient outcomes have already been demonstrated through the use of this data base. Over 1100 facility in the United States contribute to the growing data base, which now is used to show the economic implications of various levels of nurse staffing. For up-to-date information on NDNQI, enter NDNQI into the search field at http://nursingworld.org/MainMenuCategories/

QUALITY IMPROVEMENT

QI is based on the philosophy that improving the quality of health care is a never-ending process—what's considered acceptable quality today may be substandard tomorrow, especially if you consider modern advances such as diagnostic and treatment modalities, electronic information management, and new technologies.

> **RULE** At a basic level, QI studies aim to answer the question, "How can we apply the most up-to-date evidence to improve outcomes from a cost, quality-of-life, and consumer-satisfaction perspective?"

IOM and QSEN competencies stress that you must be able to participate in learning and research activities as much as feasible.[1,3] While you may not have the knowledge to do research projects, the following section helps you to determine what contributions you can make toward research, QI, and EBP.

RESEARCH AND EVIDENCE-BASED PRACTICE

EBP—moving from traditional approaches ("we do it this way because we've always done it this way") to evidence-based approaches ("we do it this way because the most up-to-date studies support that this is the best way to do it") is the cornerstone of QI.[5] Think about the implications of the following example:

EXAMPLE

Traditionally, we taught that mouth care must be done for hygiene and to prevent problems in the mouth. Research shows that poor mouth care can result in microbes colonizing the oropharynx, which then leads to pneumonia. Evidence tells us that if we don't follow strict guidelines for giving oral hygiene, we put patients at risk for deadly *pneumonia*.[6,7]

Keep in mind that EBP means more than simply "applying research." It means integrating the *best research* with *expert opinions* and *patient values* to achieve the best outcomes.[8]

Applying research to practice requires a lot of knowledge and experience. Before you apply research, you must have a good understanding of the answers to the following questions.

- What did they study and why (what was the point?)
- How did they study it (e.g., what was the study design, the number of participants, and how did they collect the data?)
- What literature did they cite?
- What were the findings?
- What are the implications of these findings?
- How does this study apply to the clinical setting where I work?

Research is often complex. If you're struggling with the answers to the above question, ask for help from your educator, mentor, or manager.

Two Good Evidence-Based Practice Web Sites

- **Agency for Health Care Research and Quality (AHRQ),** the lead Federal agency charged with translating research findings to improve the quality, safety, efficiency, and effectiveness of clinical practices: http://www.ahrq.gov
- **The Academic Center for Evidence-Based Practice (ACE),** a university-based center aiming to advance cutting-edge, state-of-the-art EBP, research, and education within an interdisciplinary context: http://www.acestar.uthscsa.edu/

Reflective Practice

Developing reflective practice—making it a habit to make time to think about how your patients are responding to your care and what you could do to improve—is not only good for patients, it's a powerful way to learn. Clinical settings are dynamic, changing, and spontaneous. No two days are the same, and each new day brings new lessons. When you have a challenging event, make time to reflect and honestly answer questions like the below. You will gain new insights and skills to help you be more confident the next time you're faced with similar situations.

Reflective Practice—Evaluating Challenging Events

- What happened?
- Why did it happen?
- What was I thinking at the time?
- What was I feeling?
- What was the worst thing about this experience?
- What was the best thing about this experience?
- What lessons did I learn from this experience?
- What will I do differently if this happens again?

Consumer Satisfaction—Maximizing Value

Evaluation gives us the feedback needed to assess consumer satisfaction and maximize the value of health care delivery. To improve and succeed as health care providers, we must consider both the needs and wants of consumers. Consider Box 6.2, which shows the types of outcomes to study to evaluate consumer satisfaction and demonstrate nurses' value.

Examining How Health Care Systems Affect Outcomes

To identify strategies to manage problems and achieve the best patient outcomes, you must look at how health care delivery systems are organized and how they all come together to affect patient care and outcomes. For example, if you work on a

---

Box 6.2 | **Improving Care and Maximizing Value**

To improve care and maximize value, gathering, analyzing, and reporting data on the following health status outcomes is critical.

- **Quality of life:** Sense of well-being, whether depression is present, success of pain management.
- **Functional status:** Ability to work, be independent, and do favorite activities.
- **Patient satisfaction:** Convenience, efficiency, and cost of care; sense that staff is attentive and sees each person as an individual.
- **Compliance measures:** Things done to help patients comply with treatment plan.
- **Impact of patient teaching:** Ability to manage own care after teaching has been done.

unit that has problems with delivery of linens, the worst situation these may create is not necessarily patients who are unhappy about their bedding. The worst problem may be wasted nursing time, as nurses spend their valuable time trying to find (or borrow) linens. Valuable nursing time is lost, and things that need to be done by nurses are omitted or done in a hurried way.

RULE   Patient outcomes—whether or not patients are safe and satisfied—are greatly affected by how care delivery systems interact with one another. For example, patients are directly affected by whether the dietary, pharmacy, and nursing departments come together to give essential nourishment and treatments in a timely way.

Three Types of Evaluation: Outcome, Process, and Structure

To ensure thorough monitoring of health care practices, QI studies consider three types of evaluation:

1. **Outcome Evaluation:** Studies the results or outcomes of care. (e.g., Were outcomes achieved within desired timeframes? Are people satisfied with care?)
2. **Process Evaluation:** Studies how the care was given. (e.g., Were assessments and interventions performed consistently and in a timely way?)
3. **Structure Evaluation:** Studies the setting in which the care takes place. (e.g., Were the physical environment, staffing patterns, and organization communication practices adequate for efficient care management?) Considering all three types of evaluation—outcome, process, and structure—provides a comprehensive examination of care management.

Box 6.3 shows example questions for all three types of studies.

Box 6.3   **Examples of Questions to Ask for Three Types of Quality Improvement Studies**

- **Outcome Evaluation (focus on results):** How many of our patients undergoing emergency bowel surgery experience an infection severe enough to delay discharge?
- **Process Evaluation (focus on how care was given):** At what point was each of our patients undergoing emergency bowel surgery first given antibiotics?
- **Structure Evaluation (focus on setting):** In what setting were antibiotics given to each of our patients undergoing emergency bowel surgery (e.g., emergency department, operating room, medical–surgical floor)?

Staff Nurses' Responsibilities

Staff nurses are accountable for participating in QI (usually for collecting data and tracking outcomes). Although QI studies may seem long and complicated, they're not only crucial to improving outcomes, they also focus on how to make your job easier and more efficient. These studies may make your next experience as a patient (or your family's next experience as a patient) better.

As a nurse who is "on the front line" with patients, you can make a valuable contribution to QI:

- **Get involved and think analytically about your practice.** As a nurse, you spend the most time with patients. If you see human problems or problems with hospital policies or procedures, report them to your supervisor.
- **Remember that how you document is important.** The records you create through ongoing documentation provide the basis for research that can benefit both health care consumers and nurses. If you're asked to do extra documentation for the purpose of these studies, realize that the information gained from the records is essential to improving quality.
- **Work on your professional improvement.** Reflect on how you can be more organized and prepared to meet your patients' needs. Be creative—think of ways you can overcome your limitations. For example, identify gaps in your knowledge and skills and ask your instructor, mentor, or manager for suggestions on what you can do to improve.

Examining Mistakes, Infections, and Injuries

In the last chapter, we addressed the importance of nursing surveillance, identifying and correcting dangerous situations, and building safety nets. Here, we address formal studies that happen after incidents of errors, injuries, and infection transmission. The aim of these studies is to identify comprehensive prevention strategies. For example, cases of unanticipated death or loss of function associated with a hospital-acquired infection will be handled as major errors that qualify as sentinel events (Box 6.4).

As a nurse—the one who spends the most time with patients—you're in the best position to identify when there are system problems that increase the risk of errors (e.g., when there are look-alike or sound-alike drugs). Stay alert for error-prone situations. Error prevention is *everyone's responsibility*. When mistakes happen, look for the root cause—the main underlying cause or contributing factors. For example, if someone gives a wrong medication, there could be many causes (e.g., lack of knowledge, poorly marked bottles, stress from work overload, or fatigue from working overtime). Box 6.5 summarizes three ways to prevent mistakes.

RULE   **EBP stresses the importance of keeping patients safe by looking for the root (main) cause of errors.** Move from a "culture of blame" (where workers hide mistakes due to fear of punitive actions) to a "culture of safety" (where high priority is given to reporting mistakes, identifying systems that are error prone, and working together to develop systems that keep patients safe).

Box 6.4	**Descriptions of Sentinel Event, Near Miss, and Hazardous Condition**

- **Sentinel event.** An unexpected incident that involves death or serious physical or psychological injury or the risk thereof. *Serious injury* specifically includes loss of limb or function. The phrase "or the risk thereof" means any variation from the usual process of care; that if it happens again, there is a significant chance of causing a serious adverse outcome. For example, a break in procedures that causes nurses to omit checking that the correct leg is marked for amputation and the wrong leg is removed. The term *sentinel* is used because of its relationship to a sentinel guard— a soldier who stands guard to keep his people safe. Sentinel events are so serious that they signal the need for immediate investigation to warrant care and ensure they don't happen again.
- **Near miss.** Anything that happens during the process of care that didn't affect the outcome, but for which a reoccurrence carries a significant chance of a serious adverse outcome. For example, if a physician almost operates on the wrong site, but this is caught just in time, it's a near miss. Near misses are considered sentinel events, but they may not be reviewed by the JCAHO under its Sentinel Event Policy.
- **Hazardous condition.** Any set of circumstances (exclusive of the disease or condition for which the patient is being treated) which significantly increases the likelihood of a serious adverse outcome.

Data from *http://www.jointcommission.org/sentinel_event.aspx*

Box 6.5	**Three Ways to Prevent Mistakes**

Although studies show that most mistakes result from basic flaws in the way the health system is organized, we all share accountability for ensuring patient safety:

1. Pay attention to things that you're doing that may create risks for errors.
2. Report systems that fail to adequately protect patients (e.g., let the risk management department know if you think of a potential change in a policy or procedure that could reduce chances for human error).
3. Empower your patients by teaching them what to expect and letting them know that the main thing they can do to prevent mistakes is to become actively involved in managing their own care.

CRITICAL THINKING AND CLINICAL REASONING EXERCISES

 Quality Improvement, Research and Evidence-Based Practice, Examining Errors, Infections, and Injuries

Example responses are provided at the end of the book (page 211).

Part One: Quality Improvement, Research and Evidence-Based Practice

1. In five sentences (or phrases) or less, explain why QI studies are important.
2. Why is it important to consider outcome, process, and structure when performing QI studies?
3. Fill in the following blanks using the following words: values, results, more, best, opinions, integrating outcomes
   EBP means (a) _____ than doing research. It means (b) _____ the (c) _____ of the (d) _____ of *research* with *expert* (e) _____ and *patient* (f) _____ to achieve the best (g) _____.

Part Two: Examining Errors, Infections, and Injuries

1. Explain the terms sentinel event, a near-miss, and a hazardous condition.
2. What is the root cause of the error in the scenario in Box 6.6?

Box 6.6   Scenario

What is the Root Cause of this Medication Error?

It's a busy evening and nurse working on a rehabilitation unit goes into a room to give a medication via a feeding tube. Following required policies and procedures, he makes sure that he has the correct patient and medication. When he goes to crush the pills, he doesn't have a pill crusher in the room. He goes back to the medication room and grabs the pill crusher. He returns to the room, crushes the pills, and begins to administer the pills through the tube. As he looks at the patient, he realizes that he came back to the wrong room and therefore had begun to give the medication to the wrong patient.

Try This on Your Own

With a peer or in a group:

1. Find a research article on a topic that interests you, then answer the following questions:
   - What did they study and why (what was the point?)
   - How did they study it (e.g., what was the study design, the number of participants, and how did they collect the data?)
   - What literature did they cite?
   - What were the findings?
   - What are the implications of these findings?
   - How does this study apply to the clinical setting where I work?
2. Discuss how you might use the information posted on Health care Research and Quality Web Site (http://www.ahrq.gov/), where you can find a wealth of information for consumers (e.g., how to quit smoking and assess health plans) and clinicians (e.g., practice guidelines and information on outcomes and effectiveness of clinical practices). Pick a few topics that interest you and see what you can learn.
3. Discuss how the links to Patient Safety Indicators posted at http://www.qualityindicators.ahrq.gov/ can impact your care practices.
4. Address how you might use the nursing process summary on the first page as a clinical guide.
5. In a personal journal, with a peer, or in a group, discuss the implications of the following *Voices* and *Think* About It entries.

Voices

New Issue Require New Thinking
The significant problems we face today cannot be solved at the same level of thinking we were at when we created them.

—Albert Einstein

Holistic and Complementary Therapies Improve Outcomes
Improving quality means considering all aspects of health care, including considering whether holistic and complementary therapies can improve results and reduce the need for treatments such as medications. For example, music therapy has been used to help children with cerebral palsy improve balance, to help stroke survivors learn how to walk again, and to help women in labor feel less pain. Music therapy can make the difference between withdrawal and awareness, between isolation and interaction, between chronic pain and comfort—between demoralization and dignity.[9]

—American Music Therapy Association

Think About It

Making Time to Reflect Helps Avoid Stamping Out Fires

If you feel like you spend too many days "stamping out fires" at work, maybe you aren't taking enough time to reflect on your practice and identify the changes you need to do to make things run smoothly.

Dietary and Housekeeping Are Your Job

Don't allow yourself to fall into the "it's not my job" mentality. If there's a problem that's delaying or compromising patient care—whether it's insufficient linens, meal trays that are consistently late, or transport people who come ill-equipped to take patients for studies—it is your job to be sure that these problems are addressed. Avoid "Band-Aid solutions," ones that are quick fixes only (e.g., constantly borrowing linens or taking your time to call the dietary department about the same problem). Rather, report these types of problems to your supervisor so that department leaders can work together to address key issues.

This Chapter and NCLEX

- Questions that focus on evaluation are complex and require in-depth analysis and interpretation. Take your time and read keywords carefully to be sure you understand what's being asked. For example, evaluation questions tend to be written something like, "Which comment (behavior) indicates the client understands or does not understand the procedure (or diet or illness?)."
- For pharmacology questions, expect to be asked how to evaluate whether the medication has worked. (e.g., What data would tell you that the antibiotic has achieved the intended therapeutic effect?)
- When a question asks about evaluating care, look for an answer that addresses assessing the patient's RESPONSE.
- If a procedure is described, think about whether it's being done CORRECTLY or INCORRECTLY.
- When the stem of the question asks about what further teaching is necessary, this indicates the client has not met the goal.

Key Points

- Careful, deliberate, and detailed evaluation of various aspects of patient care is the key to excellence in nursing.
- In context of *nursing process*, evaluation usually refers to determining the effectiveness of an individual plan of care. (i.e., Did the patient achieve the outcomes in a timely, efficient way?)
- In context of *quality improvement*, evaluation refers to ongoing studies of groups of patients to examine the effectiveness of care delivery practices.
- Comprehensive QI studies evaluate outcomes (results), process (how care was given), and structure (the setting in which care was given).

- QI requires examining how health care delivery systems interact and impact on patient outcomes.
- As a nurse, you're in a great position to identify when there are system problems that increase the risk of errors. Stay alert for error-prone situations and report them to your manager.
- You're responsible for improving your own ability to care for patients and for recognizing and reporting problems related to other departments (e.g., dietary and pharmacy). Collaborate with peers and others to identify and develop safety nets that prevent errors or catch them early.
- Scan this chapter for important rules, maps, and diagrams highlighted throughout, then compare where you stand in relation to the expected learning outcomes in the chapter opener (page 189).

References

1. Institute of Medicine. *The Future of Nursing: Leading change, advancing health.* Retrieved February 1, 2012, from http://www.nap.edu/catalog/12956.html
2. Institute of Medicine. (2000). *To err is human: Building a safer health system.* Washington, DC: National Academies Press. Retrieved February 5, 2012, from www.nap.edu/openbook.php?isbn=0309068371
3. Quality and Safety Education for Nurses. *Quality and safety competencies.* Retrieved February 5, 2012, from http://www.qsen.org/competencies.php
4. American Nurses Association. (2010). *Nursing scope and standards of performance and standards of clinical practice* (2nd ed.). Silver Springs, MD: nursesbooks.org
5. Alfaro-LeFevre, R. (2011). *Critical thinking, clinical reasoning, and clinical judgment: A practical approach* (5th ed.). Philadelphia, PA: Saunders–Elsevier.
6. Gopalan, T. (2011). Poor Oral Health can Lead to Pneumonia in Dementia Patients. *Senior Health News.* Retrieved February 5, 2012, from http://www.medindia.net/news/Poor-Oral-Health-Can-Lead-To-Pneumonia-In-Dementia-Patients-84406-1.htm
7. American Association of Critical Care Nurses. (2010). *Practice alert: Oral care for patients at risk for ventilator-associated pneumonia.* Retrieved February 5, 2012, from http://www.aacn.org/wd/practice/content/oral-care-practice-alert.pcms?menu=practice
8. Krugman, M., Habel, M., & Schultz, J. (2011). *Follow the evidence to up-to-date.* Retrieved February 5, 2012, from http://ce.nurse.com/ce359-60/follow-the-evidence-to-uptodate-practice/
9. American Music Therapy Association. Retrieved February 3, 2012, from the AMTA Web site: http://www.musictherapy.org/

EXERCISE 1.1

1. **a.** interchangeably. **b.** manage. **c.** *critical thinking.* **d.** broad.

2. **a.** *Assessment* involves examining and interviewing the patient to determine health status. During *Diagnosis*, you analyze patient information and identify the problems requiring nursing or medical treatment. In *Planning*, the expected outcomes—expected results—are determined, and the treatment plan is developed and recorded. In *Implementation*, you put the plan into action. Finally, in *Evaluation*, you assess the patient to decide whether the patient achieved the expected outcomes and modify or terminate the plan as indicated. **b.** The following characteristics of nursing process promote safe, effective clinical reasoning: purposeful, organized, systematic, humanistic, dynamic and cyclic, proactive, evidence-based, outcome-focused, cost-effective, intuitive, logical, reflective, creative improvement-oriented, and recorded in standard ways. **c.** While physicians focus on correcting and preventing problems with organs and system function, the nursing process focuses on the whole person—preventing and correcting problems with independence, human functioning, and sense of well-being.

3. Use of the nursing process is required by national practice standards; it provides the basis for questions on state board exams; it promotes safe, effective clinical reasoning; courts examine patient records to determine use of nursing process.

4. The problems identified in *Diagnosis* are based on the information collected during *Assessment*. The outcomes identified during *Planning* are based on the problems determined in *Diagnosis*. The interventions used in *Implementation* are based on the outcomes identified during *Planning*. *Diagnosis* depends on accurate assessment data.

5. If he's good at *Diagnosis*, he must be good at *Assessment*, because *Diagnosis* depends on accurate *Assessment*.

6. Assess the patient's health status (e.g., vital signs, incision, pain level).

7. Make a poster addressing the top 10 issues. Post it at the nurses' station or lounge; have a conference on the importance of meeting patients' expectations; give patients short evaluation forms to evaluate satisfaction with their nursing care (nurses are more likely to pay attention to patient expectations if they are evaluated by them).

EXERCISE 1.2

1. **a.** complex. **b.** mind.

2. Personal critical thinking indicators (Box 1.6) correspond with the top circle of the 4-Circle CT Model. Boxes 1.7 and 1.8 correspond with the other three circles.

3. You need to apply the knowledge listed in Box 1.7 to accomplish the intellectual skill in Box 1.8. However, simply having knowledge (Box 1.7) does not indicate critical thinking. It's the ability to *apply* knowledge that indicates critical thinking.

EXERCISE 2.1

Part One

1. **a.** Tell me how you're feeling. **b.** How was your dinner? **c.** How do you feel about being here? **d.** Describe what you're feeling; tell me how you're feeling.

2. **a.** So, you've been sick off and on for a month. What do you mean by sick off and on? **b.** You feel like nothing ever goes right for you. What's been happening? **c.** You have a pain in your side that comes and goes—can you explain more? **d.** You've had a funny feeling for a week. What do you mean by funny?

3. **a.** C; **b.** E; **c.** S; **d.** L; **e.** O; **f.** C; **g.** S; **h.** L; **i.** O; **j.** L; **k.** E.

4. **d.** How do you feel about feeding Susan? **h.** How would it be if your family visited? **j.** How do you feel about practicing more?

Part Two

1. **a.** You have a lot of ground-in dirt here. What's it from? **b.** I feel a lump on the back of your head. How did it happen? Does it hurt when I touch it? **c.** Your breathing is a little fast. How do you feel? **d.** Your eye seems inflamed. How does it feel?

2. **a.** Show me where (and examine that area). Is there anything you think causes it? **b.** Show me where (and examine that area). Tell me more about how it feels. **c.** That's a common symptom of infection. Let's get a urine sample (and examine it). **d.** Where do you feel this bloating? Your stomach? Ankles? Where? (and examine the area).

3. **c.**

EXERCISE 2.2

Part One

1. 51 years old, no pain, feels better, feels relieved, denies being weary.

2. Lab study results, talking slowly, frequent sighing, vital signs.

Part Two

1. All the data listed under Part One, numbers 1 and 2.

2. Physical condition seems to be improving. He is more comfortable. Seems weary/tired.

Part Three

1. **Certainly valid**: Laboratory studies, talking slowly, frequent sighing. **Probably valid**: 51 years old, no pain, feels better, vital signs, weary/tired. **Probably valid**: Weary/tired.

2. Compare age with birth date. Ask probing questions to clarify comfort state (Are you sure you don't have any discomfort?). Look for nonverbal signs of discomfort (e.g., rubbing hand on chest). Spend quality time with him discussing how he feels physically and psychologically. Recheck vital signs.

EXERCISE 2.3

1. You need to do both to promote recognition of both nursing and medical problems.

2. Body systems: **Resp**: 5, 6, 8, 10, 13, 14. **Card**: 6. **Circ**: 6, 15. GI: 9. **Neuro**: none listed. **GU**: none listed, although you might have chosen to put 11 (childbirth) here. **Skin**: None listed. Holistic nursing model: (this organizes data according to Functional Health Patterns, but you may have chosen another model) **Nutritional–Metabolic**: 5, 6, 9, 10, 11, 13, 14, 15. **Elimination**: None listed. **Activity-Exercise**: 3, 8. **Cognitive- perceptual**: None listed. **Sleep-rest**: 8. **Self-perception–self-concept**: 11 **Role-relationship**: 2, 3, 7. **Sexual–reproductive**: 1, 2. Coping Stress: 10, 12. **Value–belief**: 4.

3. You should think about how you can gain the missing information.

EXERCISE 2.4

1. **a.** N; **b.** A; **c.** N; **d.** A; **e.** A; **f.** N; **g.** A; **h.** A; **i.** N; **j.** A

EXERCISE 3.1

1. *Diagnostic reasoning* is the process of making a diagnosis (how to analyze the information you gathered during *assessment* to identify actual and potential health problems). Diagnostic reasoning is an important part of clinical reasoning because you must identify actual and potential problems in order to develop a plan to prevent and manage them.

2. *Issues* are less clearly defined than *diagnoses*, which are very specific and clearly defined based on evidence.

3. *Diagnosis* implies there's a problem that requires qualified treatment. If you make a diagnosis, you must be willing to be accountable for (a) being sure that you're qualified to treat it, and (b) initiating treatment. If you're unsure what the problem is, you're accountable for reporting it to a qualified professional.

4. *Detecting and managing risks* is the key to preventing and managing health problems.

5. Ask your supervisor or instructor whether there is a list of recommended terms. These are the terms you must use. Also review the *Do Not Use List* (these are usually abbreviations that may not be understood by others).

6. The PPMP model focuses on predicting potential complications and monitoring and intervening early-to-prevent complications. *Failure to rescue* is a term used when nurses fail to recognize when a patient is showing signs and symptoms of severe complications. Signs and symptoms can be subtle. *Nursing surveillance*—closely paying attention to patients' signs and symptoms can avoid *failure to rescue* incidents and keep patients safe.

EXERCISE 3.2

1. **a.** knowledge; experience; dialogue. **b.** qualified. **c.** domain; practice; accountability; referring

2. **a.** risk factor. **b.** potential problem. **c.** diagnosis. **d.** diagnose. **e.** accountable. **f.** medical domain. **g.** nursing domain. **h.** outcome. **i.** human response. **j.** life processes. **k.** definitive diagnosis. **l.** definitive interventions. **m.** medical diagnosis. **n.** competency. **o.** being qualified. **p.** signs. **q.** rule out. **r.** symptoms. **s.** nursing diagnosis. **t.** multidisciplinary problem..

3. The following describe nursing problems: b, d, f

4. **a.** What medications is he taking and do any of them predispose him to bleeding? **b.** Complications: internal cranial bleeding, bleeding, or infection at the laceration site. **c.** Assessments for complications of internal cranial bleeding: monitor for headache or problems with mental status, Assessments for complications of leg laceration: monitor for increased pain, bruising, swelling, redness, or warmth at the laceration site.

5. *Dehydration* related to *fever* and *poor fluid intake* as evidenced by *poor urine output* and *feeling weak*.

EXERCISE 4.1

Part One

1. Promote communication, direct care, and documentation; provide a record that can be used for evaluation and research; provide insurance companies with a record of care requirements.

2. Expected outcomes (e.g., dresses self without assistance by discharge); actual and potential problems (e.g., Self-Care Deficit: Dressing); specific interventions (e.g., have patient practice buttoning clothing three times a day); evaluation/progress notes (e.g., able to button and unbutton clothing with minimal help).

3. Patient's perception of priorities, understanding of the whole picture of problems, patient's prognosis and overall health status, expected length of stay or contact, presence of clinical guidelines or critical paths related to specific situation.

4. Severe dyspnea. Severe breathing problems are top priority unless the patient is hemorrhaging.

5. Knowing the overall discharge outcomes helps you decide which problems need to be given a high priority in order to be ready for discharge in a timely fashion.

Part Two

1. Outcomes are used to direct interventions, motivate patients and caregivers, and evaluate progress.

2. Outcome, indicator, goal, objective.

3. Outcome and indicator.

4. **a.** Report the problems to whoever is responsible for achieving the outcome. **b.** Develop and initiate a plan of care to treat the problems.

5. All nurses are responsible for detecting and reporting patients who may require case management (i.e., patients who may require extra resources to achieve the expected outcomes in a timely manner).

Part Three

1. Measurable verbs help everyone to stay focused on observable data that will let you know how well the patient is progressing toward outcome achievement. Examples: walk, explain, wash.

2. **Subject**: Who is the person expected to achieve the goal? **Verb**: What actions must the person take to achieve the goal? **Condition**: Under what circumstances is the person to perform the actions? **Performance Criteria**: How well is the person to perform the actions? **Target Time**: By when is the person expected to be able to perform the actions?

3. The following are incorrect. **a.** The verb isn't measurable. **c.** Nonspecific. How will we measure what is meant by "will improve"? **f.** No time frame listed; verb isn't measurable and observable. **i.** Verb isn't measurable.

4. **a.** Will demonstrate healthy-looking gums, without redness or irritation by Jan 15. **b.** Will not demonstrate signs and symptoms of Impaired Skin Integrity in the rectal area and area will be kept clean. **c.** Will be able to communicate basic needs through use of flash cards and through an interpreter when required.

5. SMART stands for **S**pecific, **M**easurable, **A**greed upon by all parties, **R**ealistic, **T**imebound.

Part Four

1. c, p
2. a
3. c
4. c, p.

EXERCISE 4.2

Part One

1. Classifying interventions into direct and indirect interventions allows you to examine nursing activities and time spent in direct contact with patients and activities and time spent performing activities on behalf of the patient but away from the patient (e.g., analyzing lab studies).

2. See = What must be assessed or observed related to the intervention; do = what must be done; teach = what must be taught or reinforced; record = what must be recorded related to the intervention.

3. What can be done about the cause(s) of this problem? What can be done to help this specific person achieve this specific outcome?

4. **Answer the following questions**: How reliable is the evidence that supports that the intervention(s) I plan to use is likely to work? How likely are we to see the desired

response in this particular patient and situation? What is the worst thing that can happen if this intervention is performed, and how likely is it to happen? What measures can we take to minimize the chances of causing harm? What could happen if we do nothing about this problem or these risk factors?

Part Two

1. Monitor skin integrity, especially over bony prominences, with each position change. Post at bedside a schedule for turning every 2 hours, enlisting the client's maximum participation. Keep an air mattress on the bed. Ensure adequate vitamin C and protein intake. Keep sheets clean, dry, and unwrinkled.

2. Preoperatively: Determine patient and family knowledge of coughing and deep breathing with incisional splinting. Teach as indicated and have patient return demonstration. Postoperatively: Monitor for incisional pain and medicate pm before pain is too intense. Teach the importance of asking for pain medication before pain is severe, changing positions, ambulating early, and coughing and deep breathing. Record pain level after medication is given. Record breath sounds every 4 hours. Help client to cough and deep breath every 2 hours the day of surgery and first postoperative day.

3. Monitor daily bowel movements. Teach the relationship between exercise, diet, fluid intake, and bowel elimination. Develop a plan to increase roughage and fluid intake and to increase exercise gradually (e.g., using stairs instead of elevator).

Part Three

1. PC: Extravasation, phlebitis, thrombus formation, fluid overload, infection. Plan: Follow hospital policies or standards for care of IV therapy. Monitor vital signs every 4 hours. Monitor IV site for signs and symptoms of infection, extravasation, phlebitis, thrombus every 4 hours. Instruct patient to report discomfort or swelling at IV site.

2. PC: Hypoglycemia/hyperglycemia. Plan: Follow hospital policies or standards for care of diabetics. Record daily caloric intake. Record blood sugars every 4 hours. Instruct patient to report symptoms of dizziness or "feeling funny" in any way.

3. PC: Infection, blockage of the catheter, bleeding. Plan: Follow hospital policies and standards for Foley catheter care. Monitor temperature every 4–8 hours. Monitor urine color, odor, and amount. Record intake and output every 8 hours. Monitor urinary meatus for drainage or bleeding. Instruct patient to report catheter or bladder discomfort.

Part Four

Expected outcomes, actual and potential problems, specific interventions, evaluation/progress notes.

EXERCISE 5.1

Part One

1. Standard hand-off tools help you get organized, prevents omissions of important information, and promotes dialogue and critical thinking between care givers.

2. Hand-offs are used whenever care passes from one nurse to another or when calling physicians to report concerns.

Part Two

1. competent, authority, selected, situation, accountability

2. task, worker, communication, teaching, supervision

3. **a.** See Figure 5.2. **b.** You're responsible for ensuring that your worker is capable of completing the task in each particular situation. You're also responsible for teaching the worker if teaching is indicated.

4. First and foremost, *monitor the patients*, assessing results and asking them how it's going. Supervise workers by touching base with them frequently. Be sure they know you're responsible for assessing the patient directly. If they know you will assess the patient yourself, they'll be more likely to perform the task correctly.

5. **a.** No. **b.** Because it's the first time she's getting out of bed and you don't really know how she will respond.

Part Three

1. You perform a complete assessment and determine whether the patient is progressing as expected according to plan of care. For example, if the plan includes a critical path that states "chest tubes will be out by the second postoperative day," and the patient still has chest tubes, you've identified a variance in care.

2. You should do additional assessments to determine whether the delay is justified or whether actions need to be taken to improve the patient's likelihood of achieving the outcome.

3. Additional assessments and interventions that may be required for the patient to progress may be omitted, resulting in harm to the patient or delays in recovery.

4. If the patient is harmed, you may be accused of negligence. If there are delays in recovery, you may be accused of giving substandard care.

Part Four

1. You assess patients before performing interventions to determine if the interventions are still appropriate and the patients are ready. You assess after performing interventions to determine patient response.

2. Nursing surveillance, carefully monitoring patients and their environment is a key part of performing interventions.

3. Observing for error-prone situations and care omissions is an ongoing part of performing interventions.

4. A key part of performing interventions is being proactive and planning ahead to ensure safe and effective care.

5. How you perform your interventions should be guided by your efforts to promote comfort, safety, and efficiency.

6. Always getting patient agreement before performing interventions.

EXERCISE 5.2

1. Communicate care; help you and others to identify patterns; ensure evidence-based care; provide a basis for evaluation, research, and improvement of care quality; create a legal document that later may be used in court to evaluate the type of care rendered; supply validation for re-imbursement from Medicare, Medicaid, and other insurance companies for the cost of care.

2. You'll be more accurate when the information is fresh in your mind. Charting what you've done often jogs your mind to recognize when you've forgotten to do something else you should have done.

3. AIR-A: A—States she feels like she's choking, but is afraid to cough because of incisional pain. I—Instructed how to splint incision with a pillow. R—Coughed up gray mucus plug. Lungs clear. A—Stressed the importance of reporting pain to promote better breathing and coughing.

4. **a.** It's judgmental and has no supporting evidence. **b.** It has no supporting evidence—states opinion, not facts.

5. Charting policies and procedures are designed to ensure important aspects of care are communicated, keep patients safe, and protect you in case of malpractice suits.

6. You should correct according to your school or facility polices. For hand-written notes, you usually draw a line through the note, then write the word *error*, followed by your initials.

7. *Dumping syndrome* is the problems created when you enter information into the computer and never take the time to reflect on what the information indicates.

EXERCISE 6.1

Part One

1. P.

2. A.

3. N. Insulin demand is affected by increased exercise.

4. P.

5. P. Fever and heat are also signs of infection.

Part Two

Continue the plan if the patient hasn't achieved outcomes, but you haven't identified any factors that impeded or enhanced care. Modify the plan when outcomes haven't been achieved, and you've identified factors that enhanced or impeded care. Terminate the plan if the patient has achieved outcomes and demonstrates ability to care for himself.

EXERCISE 6.2

Part One

1. Information gained from these studies improves the quality and efficiency of patient care and helps identify ways of improving nurses' job satisfaction.

2. Considering all three types of evaluation—outcome (results), process (method), and structure (setting)—provides a comprehensive examination of care management.

3. **a.** more. **b.** integrating. **c.** results. **d.** best. **e.** opinions. **f.** values. **g.** outcomes.

Part Two

1. A sentinel event is unexpected incident that involves death or serious physical or psychological injury or the risk thereof. Serious injury specifically includes loss of limb or function. The phrase "or the risk thereof" means any variation from the usual process of care; that if it happens again, there is a significant chance of causing a serious adverse outcome. For example, a break in procedures that causes nurses to omit checking that the correct leg is marked for amputation and the wrong leg is removed. The term *sentinel* is used because of its relationship to a sentinel guard—a soldier who stands guard to keep his people safe. Sentinel events are so serious that they signal the need for immediate investigation to warrant care and ensure they don't happen again. A **near miss** is anything that happens during the process of care that didn't affect the outcome, but for which a reoccurrence carries a significant chance of a serious adverse outcome. For example, if a physician almost operates on the wrong site, but this is caught just in time, it's a near miss. A **hazardous condition** when a set of circumstances significantly increases the likelihood of a serious adverse outcome.

2. The root cause is the lack of a pill crusher being in the room. It interrupted the process and created likelihood of human error. As a result of this incident, the unit made a policy that all patients who needed pills crushed must have a pill crusher at the bedside.

Example Critical Pathway

TKR Day of Surgery (date)	TKR Post-op Day 1 (date)	TKR Post-op Day 2 (date)
PHYSICAL ASSESSMENT & TREATMENT		
___ Possessions labeled and secured ___ VS Q15 min ? 3 until stable, then Q1h?;4, then Q4h ___ **VS normal, Temp <101°F** ___ Lungs clear, non-productive cough, no dyspnea ___ Oxygen as ordered ___ IS, cough & deep breathing Q1h W/A ___ I/O Q Shift ___ Nausea and vomiting tolerable w or w/o meds ___ Emesis without blood ___ Wearing TEDs ___ Skin without breakdown ___ Pneumatic boots or stockings on when in bed ___ Begin CPM setting ___ IV patent, site without redness ___ **Alert and Oriented × 3, speech clear** ___ **Normal Neurovascular checks (Q2h)** ___ **Hemovac patent and vacuum intact** ___ **Hemovac drainage <500 cc in 8 hrs** ___ **Wound bandage clean, dry and intact**	___ AM care completed ___ VS Q4h ___ **VS normal, temp <101°F** ___ IS, cough & deep breathing Q1h W/A ___ Lungs clear, non-productive cough, no dyspnea ___ Oxygen saturation >92%, oxygen discontinued ___ I/O Q Shift ___ IV line converted to saline lock, site w/o redness ___ Nausea and vomiting tolerable w or w/o meds ___ Emesis without blood ___ Wearing TEDs ___ TEDs removed ? 1/2 hr, heels w/o redness ___ Skin without breakdown ___ Pneumatic boots or stockings on when in bed ___ CPM Settings ___ Measured for brace/applied (if ordered) ___ **Alert and Oriented × 3, speech clear** ___ **Normal Neurovascular checks (Q shift)** ___ Hemovac discontinued ___ Wound dsg change time: ___ Staples/suture intact ___ Wound drainage min amt, serous/serosanguinous	___ AM care completed ___ VS Q4h ___ **VS normal, temp <101°F** ___ IS, cough & deep breathing Q4h W/A ___ Lungs clear, non-productive cough, no dyspnea ___ I/O Q Shift ___ Saline lock site w/o redness ___ Wearing TEDs ___ TEDs removed ? 1/2 hr, heels w/o redness ___ Skin without breakdown ___ Pneumatic boots or stockings when in bed ___ CPM settings ___ Brace applied (if ordered) ___ **Alert and Oriented × 3, speech clear** ___ **Normal Neurovascular checks (Q shift)** ___ Wound dsg change time: ___ Staples/sutures intact ___ Wound drainage min amt, serous/serosanguinous
PSYCHOSOCIAL ASSESSMENT		
___ Oriented to room ___ Coping effectively ___ Sleeping well: □ with medication □ without medication	___ Coping effectively ___ Sleeping well: □ with medication □ without medication	___ Coping effectively ___ Sleeping well: □ with medication □ without medication
TESTS/LABS		
___ Other tests WNL	___ H&H ≥ 9/26 ___ Chem 7 WNL ___ T/K Revision cultures no growth ___ Other:	___ H&H ≥ 9/26 ___ Other: ___ Final T/K Revision cultures without growth
PAIN CONTROL/MEDICATION		
___ IV antibiotics given ___ Ice pack to surgical site ___ Pain control: □ Spinal □ Epidural □ PCA ___ Patient reported pain level ? 3 (0–10)	___ Transfusion given if ordered □ AB □ BB □ DD ___ # of transfusions ___ IV Antibiotics completed ___ □ Spinal □ Epidural □ PCA discontinued ___ Patient reported pain level ? 3 (0–10)	___ **Offer oral meds for pain 30 minutes before therapy prn** ___ Patient reported pain level ? 3 (0–10)
NUTRITION		
___ Offered liquids	___ Diet advanced and tolerated	___ No nausea or vomiting, usual diet

A portion of a clinical pathway for total knee replacement (TKR). This section of the pathway indicates the type of clinical treatment or patient care activities to be carried out during the day of surgery and on the first 2 days after surgery for a patient undergoing TKR. The accompanying pathway documentation form is used to document any variances from the pathway that occur. (Reproduced from Inova Mount Vernon Hospital, Alexandria, VA, with permission.) **Key:** T/KI, total knee; T/K, total knee; EOB, edge of bed; SAQ, short arc quad; UE, upper extremity; LE, lower extremity; TJR, total joint replacement; RK, right knee; LK, left knee; 3:1 Commode, commode used at bedside, over toilet, and as a shower chair.

ELIMINATION

___ Foley catheter in place
___ Urine clear, output ≥30 cc/hr
___ Bowel sounds present, abdomen soft

___ Foley catheter discontinued
___ Voiding QS
___ Bowel sounds present, abdomen soft

___ Voiding QS
___ Normal bowel sounds, abdomen soft

ACTIVITY & THERAPY

___ General plan & comorbidities documented
___ Trapeze in place
___ Heels elevated while in bed
___ Dangled/stood at bedside 6–12 hrs after surgery
___ Ambulate Uni-knee

___ Trapeze in place
___ Heels elevated while in bed/knee extended
___ Ambulates to bathroom (BR) with walker or crutches uses 3:1 commode ___?
___ PT/OT eval completed, Plan of Care established
___ Goals established (Outcomes/Rehab Rounds Form)
___ Evaluation same as pre-op
___ Chart reviewed

___ Trapeze removed
___ Heels elevated while in bed/knee extended
___ Dressed in gym clothes
___ OOB for 2 of 3 meals ___?
___ Ambulates to BR with walker or crutches/assist: uses 3:1 commode ___?

Instruction and practice:
___ Ankle pump.
___ Quad/glut sets

Instruction and practice:
___ Supine to sit ___?
___ Transfers to EOB ___?
___ Dangle/Stand ___?
___ Sit to stand ___?
___ OOB in chair ___?
___ Gait on level surface ___?
___ Device ___?
___ Distance ___?

Instruction and practice:
___ Supine to sit ___?
___ Transfers to EOB ___?
___ Sit to stand ___?
___ Curbs and steps ___?

Tech treatment
___ Gait on level surface ___?
___ Device ___?
___ Distance ___?
___ Toilet transfer ___?
___ Toilet hygiene ___?
___ Grooming
___ Wash UE/trunk/LE
___ Dressing (LE)
___ Dressing (UE)
___ Shoes/socks
___ Brace on/off

Exercises in gym:
___ Ankle pump, quad/glut sets ___?
___ Heelside ___?
___ Straight Leg Raise ___?
___ SAQ (right) ___?
___ SAQ (left) ___?
___ Eval for UE group ___?

Exercises in gym:
___ Ankle pumps, quad/glut sets ___?
___ Heelside ___?
___ Straight Leg Raise ___?
___ SAQ (right) ___?
___ SAQ (left) ___?
___ Abduction/adduction ___?

	Extension	HS	Sitting flexion	Quad leg
RK	?	?		
LK	?	?		

___ Endurance
___ Instruction in set up of elevated toilet seat

	Extension	HS	Sitting flexion	Quad leg
RK	?	?		
LK	?	?		

___ Endurance
___ Instruction in set up of elevated toilet seat

TKR Day of Surgery (date) _____

EDUCATION

- TJR packet given to patient
- Post do's and don'ts, exercises at bedside

Patient instructed in/demonstrates understanding of
- IS, cough & deep breathe
- Weight bearing
- Bed mobility, use of bedpan
- Pain management, PCA/CADD

DISCHARGE PLANNING

- Family Participation reinforced
- RN completes discharge outcomes form

SURGEON NOTES

Operative Note in Progress Notes

PATIENT IDENTIFICATION		
RN D or A		
RN E		
RN N or P		
PT		
OT		
CM		
Physician		
Tech		
Other		

TKR Post-op Day 1 (date) _____

EDUCATION

Patient instructed in/demonstrates understanding of
- IS, cough & deep breathe
- Ankle pump and quad/glut exercises
- Pain management
- Weight bearing
- **Family teaching scheduled for:**

DISCHARGE PLANNING

- Plan reviewed with patient/family _____
- D/C transportation identified _____
- Discharge orders confirmed

OTHER

SURGEON NOTES

- Examination as above, variances noted
- Reviewed previous day's charting
- Plan: continue pathway

TKR POST-OP DAY 1	Time	Initials
RN D or A		
RN E		
RN N or P		
PT		
OT		
CM		
Physician		
Tech		
Other		

TKR Post-op Day 2 (date) _____

EDUCATION

Patient instructed in/demonstrates understanding of
- IS, cough & deep breathe
- Pain management
- Do's and Don'ts
- Weight bearing
- Family present for teaching

DISCHARGE PLANNING

- Home equipment discussed and ordered
- Patient adhering to pathway
- Referrals completed: __ICF__ __HHC__ __OP__ Sub acute Rehab

SURGEON NOTES

- Examination as above, variances noted
- Reviewed previous day's charting
- Plan: continue pathway

TKR POST-OP DAY 2	Time	Initials
RN D or A		
RN E		
RN N or P		
PT		
OT		
CM		
Physician		
Tech		
Other		

General Plan

Knee   ❑ Right   ❑ Left   ❑ Bilateral
        ❑ Primary   ❑ Revision   ❑ Uni-compartmental

Major Releases: _____

Weight bearing status: (with walker or 2 crutches)
❑ Non-weight bearing   ❑ 25%   ❑ 50%   ❑ Full Weight Bearing as tolerated

Brace: _____

CPM _____

Anticoagulation medication: ❑ YES   ❑ NO

Diagnosis: _____

Variance From General Plan:

❑ Yes

See Variance Documentation Pathway

Day _____

Comorbidities: (Date ID/Initials)

_____ Diabetes   _____ Hypertension   _____ HF   _____ CAD
_____ Hypothyroidism   _____ Asthma   _____ BPH   _____ COPD
_____ Obesity   _____ CABG   _____

Date/Time	Pathway Day	Variance/Problem	Action Taken/Outcome	Initials

Building Healthy Workplaces and Safety and Learning Cultures[1]

1. **Uphold Healthy Workplace Standards[2]**
   - Effective communication among all staff members (includes following a code of conduct and standards of professional behavior)
   - True collaboration
   - Effective decision making
   - Appropriate staffing
   - Meaningful recognition
   - Authentic leadership

2. **Ensure a Safety Culture**
   - **Develop skilled communication** (knowing how to listen, speak, and chart effectively). Your ability to communicate well with patients, families, peers, and other professionals makes the difference between competent, efficient care—and care that's sloppy, unprofessional, and prone to errors.
   - **Keep patient safety TOP priority** (e.g., ensure proper patient identification and apply *read back* and *repeat back* rules; follow policies and procedures closely).
   - **Recognize that because we're human, mistakes WILL happen** (usually for more than one reason).
   - **Stress that reporting errors, rather than "pointing fingers," is key to detecting and preventing mistakes.** Make everyone accountable "on their toes" looking for factors that contribute to mistakes (e.g., fatigue, communication breakdowns, staffing issues).
   - **Identify human and system factors contributing to mistakes** (join forces across disciplines to develop procedures and safety nets that address all factors).

3. **Develop a Learning Culture**
   - **Make teaching and learning a key part of daily activities of your workplace** (stress this in organizational values and performance evaluations). Encourage all to create learning opportunities and share information and strategies freely.

219

- **Be approachable—promote self-esteem and confidence** (staff, teachers, and leaders should relate to learners with kindness, showing genuine interest in them as people).
- **Uphold a good team spirit** where everyone works together toward common goals in a climate of trust and respect (help learners feel that they belong to the team).
- **Tailor teaching strategies to individuals, not tasks.** Promote independent learning in a safe environment; a lot of learning happens with trial and error and self-correction.
- **Stress that** promoting research, quality improvement, and evidence-based approaches is "everyone's job."

References

1. Alfaro-LeFevre, R. (2011). *Critical Thinking Tools: Building Healthy Workplaces and Safety and Learning Cultures.* http://www.AlfaroTeachSmart.com
2. American Association of Critical Care Nurses. Healthy Work Environments Initiatives. Retrieved February 1, 2011 from: http://www.aacn.org/WD/HWE/Content/hwehome.pcms?menu=Practice&lastmenu

Key Elements of Critical Thinking in Context of ANA Standards and QSEN and IOM Competencies

---

CRITICAL THINKING

REASONING OUTSIDE THE CLINICAL SETTING (CRITICAL THINKING)	→	REASONING IN THE CLINICAL SETTING (CRITICAL THINKING and CLINICAL REASONING)

REASONING OUTSIDE THE CLINICAL SETTING (CRITICAL THINKING)

- Problem-solving, decision-making, and judgment
- Personal, family, and community safety and welfare
- Teaching-learning (classroom, online, simulated experiences)
- Teamwork and collaboration
- Test-taking
- Using and creating electronic data
- Self improvement, stress management, and health promotion
- Community safety, welfare, and improvement
- Moral and ethical reasoning
- Long-term life planning and management

REASONING IN THE CLINICAL SETTING (CRITICAL THINKING and CLINICAL REASONING)

- Diagnostic reasoning (applying nursing process to determine, prevent, and manage patient problems)[*]
- Patient-centered care[†]
- Problem-solving, decision-making, and judgment
- Patient, caregiver, and community safety and welfare[†]
- Moral and ethical reasoning
- Applying evidence-based practice[†]
- Teamwork and collaboration[†]
- Clinical teaching and learning
- Using and creating electronic medical data (informatics)[†]
- Self improvement, stress management
- Quality Improvement (improving outcomes and care delivery systems)[†]

Effective/Skilled Communication
Knowledge-Based Thinking
Evidence-Based Thinking
Standards-Based Thinking
Analytical Thinking
Creative / Imaginative Thinking
Intuitive and Logical Thinking
Collaborative Thinking
Thinking Ahead
Thinking in Action
Thinking Back (Reflective Thinking)

Partnering With Patients and Caregivers[†]
Teaching Patients and Families[†]
Assessing Systematically[*]
Clarifying Outcomes[*]
Identifying Problems, Issues, and Risks[*]
Preventing and Solving Problems[*]
Developing and Implementing Action Plans[*]
Delegating Appropriately[†]
Monitoring Progress – Evaluating Outcomes[*]
Preventing Errors – Learning From Them[†]
Improving Performance and Process[*†]

---

[*]Required by American Nurses Association Standards (2010) Nursing scope and standards of performance and standards of clinical practice. Washington, DC: American Nurses Publishing.
[†]Relates to Quality and Safety Education for Nurses (QSEN) and Institute of Medicine (IOM) competencies. (http://www.qsen.org and http://www.iom.edu)
Key Elements of Critical Thinking in Context of American Nurses Association Standards and Quality and Safety Education for Nurses (QSEN) and Institute of Medicine (IOM) Competencies. (Source: © 2011 http://www.Alfaro TeachSmart.com. No use without permission.)

DEAD ON!! A Critical Thinking and Clinical Reasoning Game

Instructions: The point of this game is to be sure that you give key parts of thinking the time and attention they require, therefore promoting thinking that's more likely to be "dead on." Get six balls and put the letters **D, E, A, D, O, N** on each one with indelible ink. Start with **the "D" ball**, and toss it to someone in the group. Ask the group to focus on answering the questions listed under **"D"** below. Once you have exhausted thoughts on **the "D" ball**, do the same for each of the remaining balls. Be sure to *stay focused* on the current ball. For example, if someone expresses *feelings* rather than *facts* with **the "D" ball**, point out that the rules are that emotions are addressed when **the "E" ball** is up for discussion.

D = Data

- What *data (facts)* do you have?
- What *other data* do you need?
- What *assumptions* have you made and what data might validate or negate them?

E = Emotions

- What emotions (gut reactions) are there (your own, others)?
- What's your intuition telling you and what data might validate or negate it?
- How are values affecting thinking (yours, others)?

A = Advantages

- What's the vision, benefit(s), and most important desired outcome(s)?
- What are the specific advantages to *others* (benefits/ outcomes)?
- What are the specific advantages to *you* (benefits/outcomes)?

D = Disadvantages

- What could go wrong (what are the risks)?
- What are the specific inconveniences/risks for *others*?
- What are the specific inconveniences/risks for *you*?
- What problems or issues *must* be addressed to get results?
- How much work will it take and do you have the necessary resources?

O = Out of the box

- Go out of the box—think of creative approaches!
- What can we do to decrease the disadvantages?
- What can we do to increase the likelihood of seeing the benefits?
- How can technology help?
- What research is there that might apply?
- What human resources are willing to help?

N = Now what?

- What problems, risks, or issues *must* be addressed?
- Who are the key stakeholders (who will be most affected)?
- What professional, community, and informal resources can help?
- What's the plan (what interventions do you need to get results and avoid risks?
- What does all this imply?
- What did we miss when addressing the other balls? (Go through each of the balls again.)

Source: R. Alfaro-LeFevre (2003). Available at: www.AlfaroTeachSmart.com. No use without permission.

Accountable. Being responsible and answerable for something. If the quality of patient care is compromised or when allegations of unprofessional, unethical, illegal, unacceptable, or inappropriate nursing conduct, actions, or responses arise, nurses must answer to patients, employers, boards of nursing, and civil and criminal court systems.

Advanced practice nurse (APN). A nurse who, by virtue of credentials (usually completion of a master's program and certification), has a wide scope of authority to act (may include treating medical problems and prescribing medications).

Advanced practice registered nurse (APRN). *See* Advanced practice nurse.

Affective domain outcomes. Measurable goals that deal with changes in attitudes, feelings, or values.

Analyze. To examine and categorize pieces of information to determine where they might fit into the whole picture.

Anticipatory. Expected or foreseen.

Assessment. The first step of the nursing process during which you gather and organize data (information) in preparation for the second step, Diagnosis.

Assessment tool. A printed or electronic form used to ensure that key information is gathered and recorded during Assessment.

Assumption. Something that's taken for granted without proof of being the truth.

Attitude. A way of acting, feeling, or thinking that shows one's disposition, opinion, etc. (e.g., a threatening attitude).

Authority. The power or right to act, prescribe, or make a final decision.

Baseline data. Information that describes the patient's health before treatment begins (start-of-care data).

Benchmark. A standard or point in measuring quality. In health care, benchmarks are determined by analyzing the data collected over a period of time.

Best practices. A term referring to ways certain problems are best prevented and managed from an outcome and cost perspective.

CareMap. *See* Critical pathway.

Care partner. *See* Unlicensed assistive personnel (UAP).

Care variance. *See* Variance in care.

Caring behavior. A way of acting that shows understanding and respect for others' ideals, values, feelings, needs, and desires.

Case management. An approach to patient care that aims to improve patient outcomes and satisfaction while reducing overall cost and length or incidence of hospital stays.

Client-centered outcome. A statement describing a measurable behavior of a client, family, or group that reflects the desired result of interventions (that the problem, or problems, are prevented, resolved, or controlled).

Client goal. *See* Client-centered outcome.

Clinical pathway. *See* Critical pathway.

Cognitive domain outcomes. Measurable goals that deal with acquiring knowledge or intellectual skills.

Competence. The quality of having the necessary knowledge and skill to perform an action in a safe and appropriate way, under various circumstances.

Critical. Characterized by careful and exact evaluation and judgment.

Critical pathway. A standard plan that predicts the course of recovery and day-by-day care required to achieve outcomes for a specific health problem within a specific time frame.

Cues. Pieces of information that prompt you to draw a conclusion about health status.

Data base assessment. Comprehensive data collected on initial contact with the patient to gain information about all aspects of the patient's health.

Data base form. *See* Assessment tool.

Defining characteristics. A cluster of cues (signs, symptoms, and risk [related] factors) often associated with a specific nursing diagnosis.

Definitive diagnosis. Most specific, most correct, diagnosis.

Definitive interventions. The most specific treatment required to prevent, resolve, or control a health problem.

Delegation. The transfer of responsibility for the performance of an activity while retaining accountability.

Diagnose. To make a judgment and identify a problem or strength based on evidence from an assessment.

Diagnosis. (1) The second step of the nursing process. (2) The process of analyzing data and putting related cues together to make judgments about health status. (3) The opinion or judgment that's drawn after the diagnostic process is completed.

Diagnostic error. When a health problem has been overlooked or incorrectly identified.

Diagnostic reasoning. A method of thinking that involves specific, deliberate use of critical thinking to reach conclusions about health status.

Direct care interventions. Actions performed through interaction with patients (e.g., helping someone out of bed, teaching someone about diabetes).

Direct data. Information gained directly from the patient.

Empathy. Understanding another's feelings or perceptions, but not sharing the same feelings or point of view (compare with Sympathy).

Etiology. Something known to cause a disease.

Evidence-based practice. Clinical practices that integrate the *best research* with *clinical expertise* and *patient values* to achieve the best outcomes. Requires knowing the strength of the evidence that supports your interventions.

Expedite. To speed up.

Focus assessment. Data collection that concentrates on gathering more information about a specific problem or condition.

Guidelines. Documents that delineate how care is to be provided in specific situations. *See* also

Protocols, Policies, Procedures, Standards, and Standards of care.

Habits of inquiry. Thinking habits that enhance your ability to search for the truth (e.g., following rules of logic).

Humanistic. *See* Caring behavior.

Indicators. Concrete, observable behaviors that can be observed to determine outcome achievement (e.g., joint movement, absence of skin redness).

Indirect care interventions. Actions performed away from the patient but on behalf of a patient or group of patients. These actions are aimed at management of the health care environment and interdisciplinary collaboration.

Indirect data. Information gained from sources other than the patient (e.g., someone's wife).

Inference. A conclusion drawn from a patient cue (or cues).

Intervention. An action performed to prevent or manage problems or to maximize comfort and human functioning.

Intuition. Knowing something without having supporting evidence.

Judgment. An opinion that's made after analyzing and synthesizing information.

Life processes. Events or changes that occur during one's lifetime (e.g., growing up, aging, maturing, becoming a parent, moving, separations, losses).

Long-term goal. An objective that's expected to be achieved over a relatively long time period, usually weeks or months.

Medical diagnosis. A problem requiring definitive diagnosis by a qualified physician or advanced practice nurse.

Medical domain. Activities and actions a physician is legally qualified to perform or prescribe.

Medical orders. Interventions ordered by a physician or advanced practice nurse to treat a medical problem.

Medical process. The method physicians use to expedite diagnosis and treatment of diseases or trauma. The medical process focuses mainly on problems with structure and function of organs or systems.

Multidisciplinary plan. A plan that's developed collaboratively by key members of the health care team (e.g., nursing, physical therapy, medicine).

Need. A requirement that, if fulfilled, reduces stress and promotes a sense of adequacy and well-being.

Nurse extender. *See* Unlicensed assistive personnel (UAP).

Nurse-prescribed intervention. An action a nurse may legally order or initiate independently.

Nursing assistant. *See* Unlicensed assistive personnel (UAP).

Nursing domain. Activities and actions a nurse is legally qualified to perform or prescribe.

Objective data. Information that is measurable and observable (e.g., blood pressure, pulse, diagnostic studies).

Outcome. The result of prescribed interventions; usually refers to the desired result of interventions (i.e., that the problem is prevented, resolved, or controlled) and includes a specific time frame for when the goal is expected to be achieved.

Palliative care. Care that alleviates pain and suffering but doesn't cure.

Patient care technician. *See* Unlicensed assistive personnel (UAP).

Policies. *See* Guidelines.

Primary care provider. The health care professional designated to be in charge of managing the patient's major medical problems (may be a physician, advance practice nurse, or physician's assistant).

Proactive. A way of thinking and behaving that accepts responsibility for one's actions and takes initiative to plan ahead to anticipate and prevent problems before they happen (comes from "act before").

Procedures. *See* Guidelines.

Prognosis. The predicted course or outcome of disease or trauma.

Protocols. *See* Guidelines.

Psychomotor outcomes. Measurable goals that deal with acquiring skills that require deliberate, specific muscle coordination to perform an activity (e.g., walking with crutches).

Qualified. Having the knowledge, skill, and authority to perform an action.

Quality care. Cost-effective health care that increases the probability of achieving desired results and decreases the probability of undesired results.

Related factor. Something known to be associated with a specific diagnosis. *See* also Risk factor.

Risk factor. Something known to cause or contribute to a specific problem (e.g., decreased vision contributes to Risk for Injury).

Risk (potential) diagnosis. A health problem that may develop if preventive actions aren't taken.

Sign. Objective data that indicate an abnormality.

Stakeholders. Those who are most affected by the plan of care, for example, patients, families, caregivers, and third-party payers.

Standard care plan. A preformulated plan that can be used as a guide to expedite development and documentation of a plan of care. *See* also Guidelines.

Standard of care. A document outlining the minimal level of routine care provided for all patients in certain situations (focuses on what will be observed in the patient to let you know the care has been given). *See* also Guidelines.

Standard of practice. A document outlining what the nurse will do in giving care in specific situations. *See* also Guidelines.

Standard of professional performance. Statements that describe a competent level of behavior in the professional role.

Standards. Authoritative statements by which the nursing profession describes the responsibilities for which its practitioners are accountable. *See* also Guidelines.

Subjective data. Information the patient or client tells the nurse during Assessment (usually charted as "Patient states. ...").

Sympathy. Sharing the same feelings as another (compare with Empathy).

Symptom. Subjective data that indicate an abnormality.

Syndrome diagnosis. A cluster of nursing diagnoses often associated with a specific situation or event.

Unlicensed assistive personnel (UAP). Someone without a license to practice nursing who is hired to assist nurses in care delivery. These individuals may have a variety of job titles (e.g., nursing assistant, nurse extender, care partner, patient care technician) and have varied job descriptions and capabilities.

Variance in care. A case in which a patient hasn't achieved activities or outcomes by the time frame noted on a critical path. A variance in care triggers additional assessment to determine whether the delay is justified or whether actions need to be taken to improve the patient's likelihood of achieving the outcome.

Index

Note: Page numbers followed by *b* indicate boxed material; page numbers followed by *f* indicate material in figures; page numbers followed by *t* indicate material in tables.

DATE DUE

COMMON MEDICAL PROBLEMS AND THEIR POTENTIAL COMPLICATIONS*

ANGINA/MYOCARDIAL INFARCTION

Dysrhythmias
Congestive heart failure/pulmonary edema
Shock (cardiogenic, hypovolemic)
Infarction, infarction extension
Thrombi/emboli formation (pulmonary emboli, stroke)
Hypoxemia
Electrolyte imbalance
Acid–base imbalance
Pericarditis
Cardiac tamponade
Cardiac arrest
    See also Kidney Disease

LUNG DISEASES (ASTHMA, COPD, ETC.)

Hypoxemia
Acid–base and electrolyte imbalance
Respiratory failure
Infection
    See also Pneumonia and Angina/Myocardial
        Infarction

PNEUMONIA

Respiratory Failure
Dehydration
Sepsis/septic shock
Pulmonary embolus
Pulmonary hypertension
    See also Angina/Myocardial Infarction

DIABETES

Hypoglycemia (diabetic shock)
Hyperglycemia (diabetic coma)
Compromised circulation—pressure and leg ulcers
Delayed wound healing
Hypertension
Eye problems (retinal hemorrhage)
Infection
Dehydration
    See also Angina/Myocardial Infarction and Kidney
        Failure

HYPERTENSION

Stroke (cerebrovascular accident—CVA)
Transient ischemic attacks (TIAs)
Hypertensive crisis
    See also Angina/Myocardial Infarction and Kidney
        Failure

KIDNEY DISEASE

Congestive heart failure
Kidney failure

Edema
Hyperkalemia
Electrolyte/acid–base imbalance
Anemia
    See also Hypertension and Urinary Tract Infection

URINARY TRACT INFECTION (UTI)

Septic shock
Kidney failure

HIV AND IMMUNOSUPPRESSION

Opportunistic infections (TB, herpes, intestinal
    organisms, etc.)
Severe diarrhea
    See also Lung Diseases and Pneumonia

FRACTURES

Bleeding (internal or external)
Bone fragment displacement
Edema/pressure points
Compromised circulation
Nerve compression
Compartment syndrome
Thrombus/embolus formation
Infection

HEAD TRAUMA

Respiratory depression
Airway occlusion
Aspiration
Bleeding (internal or external)
Shock
Brain swelling
Increased intracranial pressure
Seizures/coma
Hyper/hypothermia
Infection

OTHER TRAUMA

See Anesthesia/Surgical Invasive Procedures
    (next page)

DEPRESSION/PSYCHIATRIC DISORDERS

Reality distortion
Dehydration/malnutrition
Suicide
Violence (against self or others)
Self-protection problems
Medication side effects

*Partial list. Consult your textbooks for additional problems.

RRS1210